Risk Factors in Implant Dentistry

Simplified Clinical Analysis for Predictable Treatment

Risk Factors in Implant Dentistry

Simplified Clinical Analysis for Predictable Treatment

Franck Renouard, DDS

Private practice, Oral and Maxillofacial Surgery

Consultant
Paris V University
Paris, France

Bo Rangert, PhD, Mech Eng

Associate Professor of Biomedical Engineering
Rensselaer Polytechnic Institute
Troy, New York

Director of Clinical Research
Nobel Biocare AB
Gothenburg, Sweden

Chicago, Berlin, London, Tokyo, Paris
São Paulo, Barcelona, Moscow, Prague, and Warsaw

To Nadine, Erell, and Nolwenn
Maud, Åsa, Tora, and Elsa

First published in French by Quintessence International, Paris, 1999

Library of Congress Cataloging-in-Publication Data

Renouard, Franck.
    [Facteurs de risque et traitements implantaires. French]
    Risk Factors in Implant Dentistry : Simplified Clinical
Analysis for Predictable Treatment / Franck Renouard, Bo
Rangert.
         p.   cm.
    Includes bibliographical references.
    ISBN 0-86715-355-5
    1. Dental implants—Complications.   2. Dental implants.
 I. Rangert, Bo.   II. Title.
    [DNLM: 1. Dental implants—adverse effects.   2. Risk factors.
WU 640 R419r   1999]
RK667.I45R4613 1999
616.6'92—dc21
DNLM/DLC
for Library of Congress   99-19894
                                          CIP

© 1999 Quintessence Publishing Co, Inc

Quintessence Publishing Co, Inc
551 Kimberly Drive
Carol Stream, Illinois 60188

Printed in Germany

Foreword

In all clinical procedures that interfere with the human body, there is an element of risk. Carefully worded comments on this crucial issue must reach the patient, often repeatedly, to avoid unnecessary bodily, mental, or legal harm to the patient or those providing treatment. This requires that the clinician establish a relationship and interaction with the patient, so that his or her needs, demands, anatomy, and function can be understood and identified. Further, it is necessary to explain and visualize what is possible to achieve, based on established treatment modalities and the experience of those about to treat the patient. It is equally important to expose unrealistic expectations of the patient and amongst the patient's social surroundings.

Clinical osseointegration derives from hardware and software that together create a reconstruction system. The therapeutic capacity relies on a team effort—not only to support clinical decisions and procedures but also to provide constructive critical comments, advice, and suggestions in the individual case. Before any novel treatment procedure is considered, or if new or modified compo-

nents that lack long-term data are used, it is imperative that possible consequences of deviations from an established, documented protocol be evaluated.

Edentulism, being a serious handicap, should be treated with the utmost respect. A clinical approach should, therefore, include means to avoid or minimize complications and failures by optimizing treatment selection, efforts, and ambitions. When there is a doubt as to what to suggest or what to do it might be better to refrain from treatment at that time to allow for consultations outside the team or to refer the patient to another clinical unit.

This book is intended to show clinicians how to identify, prevent, and avoid problems in implant treatment by following logical clinical protocols.

Professor Per-Ingvar Brånemark

Preface

On June 4, 1984, a little by chance, I joined the craniofacial surgical team of Paul Tessier as assistant to Jean-François Tulasne. On June 18, 1984, in France, Dr Tulasne placed the first six Brånemark implants. During this epoch things were simple; there was one single type of implant, one single type of abutment, and only one indication: complete edentulism.

Complications began when partial edentulism and, later, single tooth loss were treated, still with one single type of implant and one single type of abutment. Soon the responsibility for the treatment was assumed by the surgeons. Because they treated many more patients than did general practitioners, the surgeons imposed their concept of osseointegration: anchorage above all.

Against this dogma and its consequences for the position and inclination of the implants, the practitioners responsible for the prostheses involved themselves in defining the precise conditions for the successful implant-supported prosthesis. The battlefield thus changed. The aim for the implant treatment became the prosthesis: The implant should therefore be placed exactly in the direction and the position defined by the waxup, leaving bone volume unconsidered. It became indispensable to complete repeated radiographic examinations to obtain surgical guides of irrefutable precision. Other problems had also appeared: proximity between implants, use of non-adapted implant diameters, insufficient number of implants, questionable prosthetic concepts with screw-retained esthetic extensions, and so on.

To meet the demands for all the clinical indications, a multitude of surgical and prosthetic components were proposed. Guided bone regeneration and bone-grafting techniques were developed to allow ideal implant placement, independent of the initial bone volume. Closer and closer collaboration between the surgical and prosthetic teams has led to the definition of protocols that are better adapted to each particular clinical situation.

At the same time, despite following scrupulous surgical and prosthetic techniques, all implant teams are confronted with a certain amount of complications. It was necessary to analyze these problems to find the reasons. Fundamental research has thus progressed, especially in the areas of biomechanics and peri-implant pathosis.

From retrospective studies of complications and failures, it became apparent that, for implant treatment, as for all other medical disciplines, 80% of the problems are found in 20% of the patients. The notion of risk patients was introduced little by little.

The goal of this book is to propose a methodology to detect these patients in advance, with the purpose of reducing or eliminating the risk for failure. As soon as a risk situation is diagnosed, it is possible to modify the treatment plan (prolong the healing time, add extra implants, reduce prosthetic extensions, etc) or to decide that implant treatment is contraindicated.

The first three chapters are devoted to the analysis of the general, esthetic, and biomechanical risk factors. Then all types of edentulism are described in chapters 4 and 5, and the safest treatment options, as well as alternative solutions, are presented for each situation. Tables summarize the limitations and the risk factors specific for each particular clinical situation.

Different surgical protocols as well as bone-related problems are approached in chapter 6. Chapter 7 examines the need for the practitioner to study communication problems with the patient. Finally, in chapter 8, complications and failures are covered in the most simple and didactic manner possible.

Writing this introduction represents both happiness, as it signifies the result of 18 months work, and, on the other hand, a feeling of sadness, as it concludes the nearly daily collaboration between Bo Rangert and me.

The prosthetic work of the clinical cases has all been performed by the referring practitioners, associated with a private practice. Thanks goes to all these colleagues, and in particular Drs Jean Michel Gonzalez and Philippe Rajzbaum, both long-time assistants at the dental surgical faculty at University of Paris V, who made the prostheses for most of the patients in this book. They also actively participated with suggestions and ideas that made it possible to realize the project.

The therapeutic team would not be complete if the laboratory technicians and radiologists were forgotten. Thanks to all of them for their active and precious collaboration.

Finally, let's not forget my partners, Drs Jean-François Tulasne (maxillofacial surgeon) and Jean-Louis Giovannoli (periodontist), without whom this book would never have been initiated.

All the drawings for the book were made by Fredrik Persson and are reproduced with the courtesy of Nobel Biocare AB.

Franck Renouard

Contents

Chapter 1

General Risk Factors

The use of implants has, little by little, been imposed on the world of dentistry. Some years ago, it was strongly suggested that the practitioners asked implant patients to sign a consent form to release the dentist from all responsibility in case of failure. Then, one day a patient in France sued his dentist for having prepared his teeth for a fixed partial denture without suggesting the implant alternative. The patient won the case. Soon it might be necessary to ask patients to sign a form indicating that they have refused implant treatment.

However, an implant prosthetic reconstruction does not offer miracles. Complications and failures are possible. The mere knowledge of the technique of implant treatment is not sufficient to eliminate all problems. The dentist has to be able to analyze a given clinical situation and evaluate its complexity.

For a long time, the identification of a risk patient has been directly related to anatomic considerations: ample bone meant a good patient and insufficient bone a bad one. Subsequent analysis of failures, step by step, has led to a better understanding of the parameters that permit a high overall treatment success rate, encompassing criteria related to health, function, and esthetics.

However, the treatment protocols have a tendency to become simpler. The use of self-tapping or large-diameter implants offers the surgeon means of treating situations that were considered restricted only a few years ago. Likewise, for the prosthetic side, the multitude of components and abutments, which may be perceived as increasingly complex, now allows the clinician to treat the majority of situations with a standardized protocol.

The difficulty with implant treatment essentially lies in the ability to detect risk patients.

A risk patient is a patient in whom the strict application of the standard protocol does not give the expected results.

For example, a smoker has a 10% higher risk of osseointegration failure. Likewise, a bruxer has an increased risk of fracturing prosthetic components. These patients should be considered risk patients. Some risk factors are relative, while others are absolute. The distinction between the two is not as clear as it might appear. However, a number of relative contraindications or one absolute contraindication should lead to a reevaluation of the original treatment plan.

	OKAY	CAUTION	DANGER
General health			
	Old infarct	Angina Coronary disease Interauricular or interventricular communication	Valvulopathies Recent infarct Severe cardiac insufficiency
		Anticoagulant treatment	Hemopathy Agranulocytosis
		Renal insufficiency	Immunodeficiency
		Diabetes	Evolving cancer
		Polyarthritic rheumatism	Hemophilia
		Anemia	Transplantation
		Scleroderma	AIDS
		Lupus	
		Respiratory insufficiency	
		Seropositivity for HIV	
		Osteoporosis	Osteomalacia
			Osteogenesis imperfecta
			Paget's disease
	Patient over 18 years	Elderly patient	Patient under 16 years
		Pregnancy	
		Alcoholism	
		Severe tabagism	
		Drug addiction	
		Cervicofacial irradiation	
Patient interrogation			
Obsessional neurosis	No	+/–	Yes
Esthetic demands	Realistic	High	Unrealistic
Availability	Yes	No	
Etiology of the edentulism			
Caries	Yes		
Trauma	Yes		
Periodontal disease		Yes	
Occlusal trauma		Yes	Yes
Extraoral examination			
Smile line (anterior edentulism)	Dental	Gingival	

Intraoral examination

	Three fingers	Two fingers	
Jaw opening	Three fingers	Two fingers	
Hygiene	Good	Poor	
Lesion, abscess, etc present	No		Yes
Intraoral palpation		Shallow vestibule	
Vestibular concavity present	No	Yes	
Interarch relations: Maxillomandibular discrepancy	No	Yes	
Vertical bone resorption	No	Yes	
Height between bone crest and opposing tooth	>7 mm	6 mm	<5 mm
Interarch distance at maximal opening	>35 mm		<30 mm
Mesiodistal distance: 1 implant 2 implants 3 implants	>7 mm >15 mm >21 mm	7 mm 14 mm 20 mm	<6 mm <13 mm <18 mm
Functional evaluation			
Bruxism/parafunction		Yes	Yes
Lateral guidance with natural teeth	Yes	No	
Natural teeth participating in proprioception	Yes	No	
Radiographic examination			
chronic lesions			
– Close to the implant zone	No		Yes
– Distant from the implant zone	Yes	Yes	
Periodontal evaluation			
Gingivitis	Yes		
"Treated" periodontitis		Yes	
Active periodontitis			Yes

Note:
The list of pathoses representing relative or absolute contraindications is not exhaustive.

Preliminary Examination

The aim of the preliminary examination before implant treatment is to identify, at an early stage, any relative or absolute contraindication. It is useless to prescribe a computerized tomographic scan if the patient is not able to open the mouth more than the width of two fingers.

The first checklist is used at the first clinical examination to find out if the patient is a good candidate for implant treatment. The definitive treatment plan, including number of implants, their dimensions, and their position, is not decided until after the final radiographic examination.

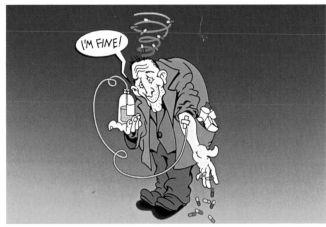

Fig 1-1 The preoperative clinical examination should enable the detection of patients in whom implant surgery is contraindicated. (Drawing by Etienne Pelissier.)

General examination

General health

Absolute medical contraindications for implant treatment are rare. The risk of a focal infection with an osseointegrated implant is very low and certainly much lower than with a devitalized tooth. However, implant surgery presents the same contraindications as any bone surgery. Therefore, it is very important to identify patients who have general pathoses (Fig 1-1) (pages 14 and 15).

The distinction between relative and absolute contradictions is not perfectly defined and should be adapted to different conditions, for example, the experience of the clinician. Certain patients who present general pathoses, such as diabetes and anemia, should be treated by a well-trained surgical team under conditions that scrupulously respect the surgical protocol, especially the strict aseptic conditions.

Notably, smoking increases the failure rate about 10% and is a contraindication for protocols such as bone regeneration or bone grafting.

Age

Implants should not be used on young patients before the end of their growth, which is approximately at 16 years for girls and 17 to 18 years for boys.

On the other hand, there is no upper age limit. However, elderly patients often present a number of general health problems, which might contraindicate surgery.

Patient psychology and motivation

Implant treatment is still not widely known by the general public. The information is generally spread by the weekly magazines or word of mouth, and not always objectively. Too often, implants are analogous to esthetic treatment. This misinformation could have a major impact on a patient's implant treatment, and it is very important to identify patients who have unrealistic esthetic demands. The higher the esthetic requirements, the more necessary it is for the patient to be cooperative and perfectly aware of the difficulties, the limitations, and the duration of the treatment.

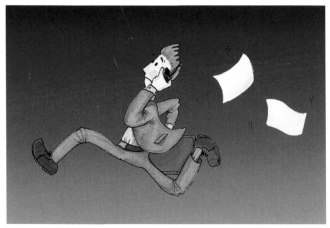

Fig 1-2 If the patient's schedule is not accommodating, it is preferable not to initiate complex treatments requiring frequent recalls, such as guided tissue regeneration, bone grafting, etc. (Drawing by Ingrid Balbi.)

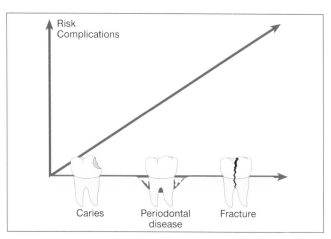

Fig 1-3 The etiology of the patient's edentulism is an indicator of the potential risk for complications of implant treatment.

Availability

Certain treatment requires frequent availability of the patient. For example, after a guided bone regeneration procedure it is necessary to verify, about every third week, at least during the first months of healing, that the membrane is not exposed. This kind of treatment might be contraindicated for patients who are very busy and not available (Fig 1-2).

Etiology of the edentulism

Often implant candidates arrive for the initial consultation and their dental history is unknown to the practitioner responsible for the treatment. However, the etiology of the edentulism is extremely important to know (Fig 1-3).

If the patient has lost the teeth to caries or trauma (sports, accident, etc), the inherent risk of implant failure is small.

If the tooth loss is related to periodontal disease, the etiologic factors of the disease must be eliminated before the implant treatment commences. Such patients should be considered to be associated with a small or moderate risk. The presence of periodontal disease has little influence on the im-

plant osseointegration process (if the implants are buried). However, the pathogenic bacteria existing in the pockets around natural teeth could infect the peri-implant tissue, leading to mucositis (inflammation of peri-implant soft tissue) and/or peri-implantitis (infectious bone loss around the implant).

If the edentulism is associated with natural teeth fractured because of bruxism or severe occlusal disorder, the patient should be considered to have a significant risk factor. Implant treatment in such cases should not be proposed unless a sufficient number of implants can be placed.

Extraoral examination

■ Smile line (Figs 1-4 and 1-5)
The position of the smile line should be noted at the first consultation. Often, a fixed implant prosthesis does not have the same esthetic opportunities as a traditional prosthesis, especially if the crest morphology indicates a possible need for guided tissue regeneration or bone grafting. For all anterior restorations, a patient who exposes a large portion of gingiva while smiling should be considered as a risk patient from an esthetic point of view (see chapter 2).

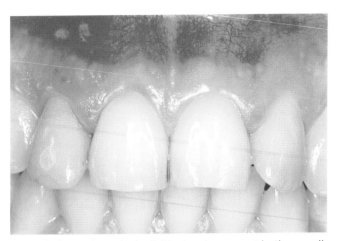

Fig 1-4 An endoperiodontal lesion is present in the maxillary right lateral incisor. The tooth is to be extracted, and an implant solution is planned.

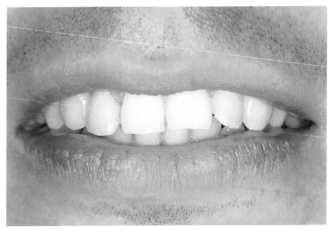

Fig 1-5 Same patient. The gingiva is not exposed during smiling, and the situation is favorable for implant placement.

Intraoral examination

■ Jaw opening (Fig 1-6)

The first thing to do before the intraoral examination is to register the jaw opening. The width of three fingers corresponds to approximately 45 mm, which represents an ideal opening. Two fingers represents the lower limit, under which it is not possible to treat the posterior regions.

■ Hygiene (Figs 1-7 and 1-8)

The evaluation of the patient's oral hygiene is not relevant for the implant treatment per se. However, attention should be paid to patients who have been edentulous for a long time. They have often forgotten the simple measures of oral hygiene. Sometimes it is necessary to adapt a treatment plan that favors simple solutions such as an overdenture, even if the bone volume is considerable.

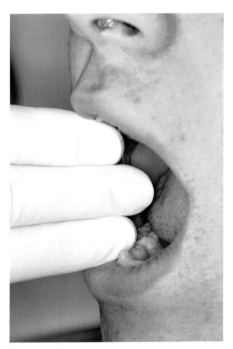

Fig 1-6 The jaw opening should be checked before the intraoral examination begins. An opening width of three fingers represents a favorable situation.

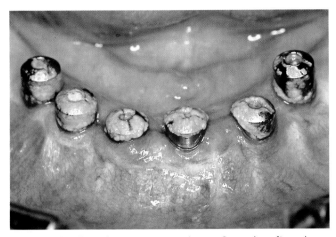

Fig 1-7 Healing abutments are shown 3 weeks after placement in a patient who had been edentulous for a long time. Such patients have often forgotten the simple measures of oral hygiene. They have to be motivated and followed with special care.

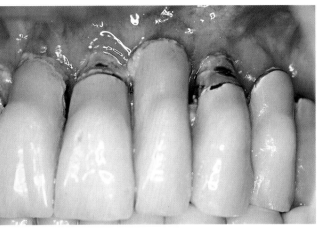

Fig 1-8 A complete-arch maxillary prosthesis is shown in an elderly patient at the 6-month follow-up. The extreme length of the prosthetic crowns is intended to compensate for the severe vertical bone resorption. This type of restoration is very difficult to clean. Patients who have difficulties maintaining rigorous oral hygiene are sometimes better off with an overdenture or a prosthesis with high abutment pillars, possibly with false gingiva, if esthetic or functional (phonetics) problems are present.

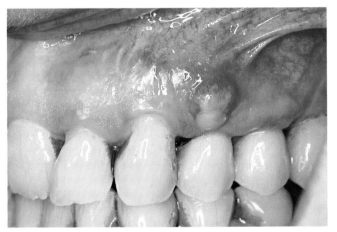

Fig 1-9 The maxillary left first premolar has been lost and should be replaced with an implant. The presence of an acute infection is a definite contraindication for immediate implant placement. Implant surgery should be delayed a minimum of 2 months. However, a period of 6 to 8 months is preferable.

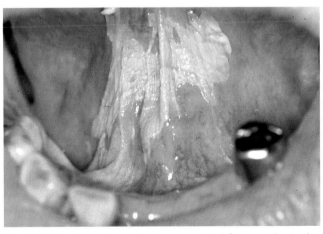

Fig 1-10 Implants have been suggested for a patient who has large areas of leukoplakia. A dermatologist should be consulted before implant therapy is initiated.

■ Presence of lesions, abscess, etc (Figs 1-9 and 1-10)

The presence of any acute infection is a temporary, absolute contraindication for placing implants. Implant surgery should not be performed before the lesion is treated and healed. Although no study exists on the subject, the clinician should be careful with patients who have mucosal lesions. A consultation with a dermatologist might be necessary.

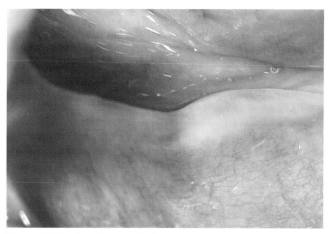

Fig 1-11 During the preliminary examination, intraoral palpation reveals knife-edged ridges, which represent a difficult situation for the surgeon. However, the precise bone morphology will not be known until after the radiographic examination.

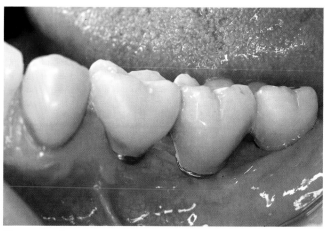

Fig 1-12 The progressive decrease of the crestal bone height is generally followed by a reduction in depth of the vestibule. This clinical situation represents a risk for the peri-implant tissue health. Because of the high attachment of the buccinator muscle, a keratinized gingival graft is not always possible.

▓ Intraoral palpation

The intraoral palpation should be used to evaluate the following:

- The sharpness of the crest. Even if this measure is imprecise, it indicates knife-edged ridges, for which bone augmentation techniques often are necessary (Fig 1-11).
- The depth of the vestibule. A shallow vestibule is often the result of substantial bone resorption; in these situations, a good esthetic result is more difficult to obtain and the hygiene will be more problematic for the patient (Figs 1-12 and 1-13).
- The presence of a vestibular concavity close to the implant sites (Figs 1-14 to 1-16).
- The anterior sinus wall, which most often bulges at the position of the maxillary premolars.

▓ Interarch relations (Figs 1-17 and 1-18)

Anteroposterior or lateral discrepancies in the maxillomandibular relations may lead to prosthetic risks. Biomechanically, this situation could be hazardous, especially in combination with functional risks, such as bruxism.

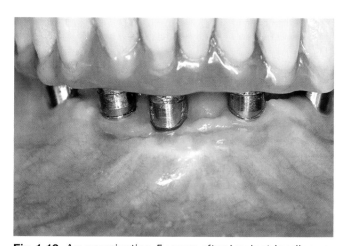

Fig 1-13 An examination 5 years after implant loading reveals the absence of the vestibule resulting from the vertical resorption of the crest. Hygiene maintenance can be difficult, especially for elderly patients. A prosthesis on high abutments offers an interesting solution in these situations. (Prostheses by Dr D. Vilbert and S. Tissier.)

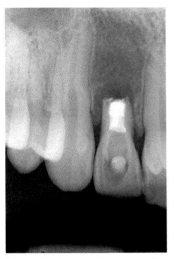

Fig 1-14 A retroalveolar radiograph reveals significant resorption at the maxillary right lateral incisor. An implant tooth replacement is planned.

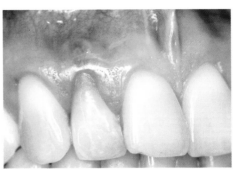

Fig 1-15 Same patient. The gingival level seems appropriate for an esthetic restoration (see chapter 2).

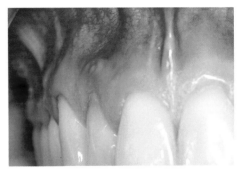

Fig 1-16 Same patient. For this esthetically demanding restoration, it is crucial that the implant be placed exactly along the axis of the prosthetic crown. Note the large concavity at the lateral incisor. Implant placement will not be possible unless a bone graft is completed first.

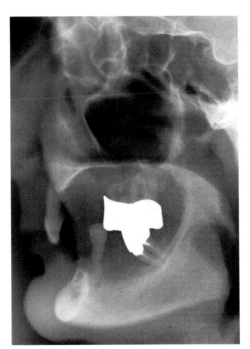

Fig 1-17 The radiographic profile of a patient before placement of implants at the mandibular symphysis reveals an anteroposterior discrepancy between the maxilla and the mandible. To limit the vestibular offset, and in spite of a sufficient volume of bone, an overdenture is indicated. (Photo by Dr G. Pasquet and Dr R. Cavezian.)

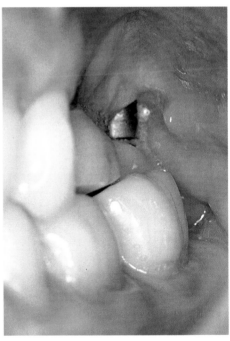

Fig 1-18 The maxillary left molars have been lost, resulting in a significant loss of bone. Two implants have been placed because of the limited bone volume available. Note the buccal position of the mandibular left second molar. The unfavorable occlusal relationship represents a functional risk (see chapter 3).

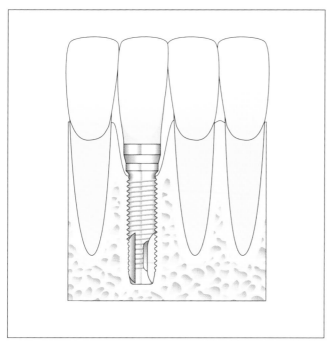

Fig 1-19 Esthetic and biologic problems are associated with placing an implant too far apically.

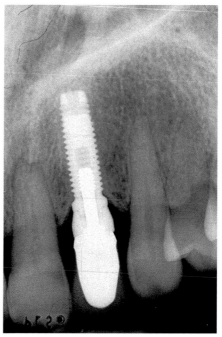

Fig 1-20 A Regular Platform implant has been used to replace the maxillary left lateral incisor. Radiographic follow-up 5 years after implant loading reveals the deep apical position of the implant relative to the line connecting the approximating cementoenamel junctions.

■ Vertical bone resorption (Figs 1-19 to 1-21)
Most often, the loss of a tooth is followed by bone loss of minor or major importance. It is necessary to evaluate the discrepancy between the bone level at the implant site and the level at the adjacent teeth. Too large a difference represents a risk to both periodontal and peri-implant tissue health and esthetics. Facing this situation, the clinician should consider reconstruction of the crest with bone regeneration or grafting before implant placement.

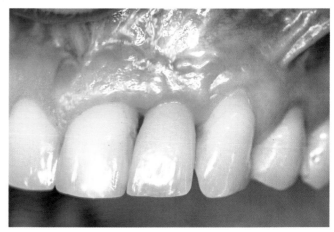

Fig 1-21 Same patient. The clinical view at the 5-year follow-up reveals the gingival recession distal to the central incisor, resulting from the deep apical position of the implant.

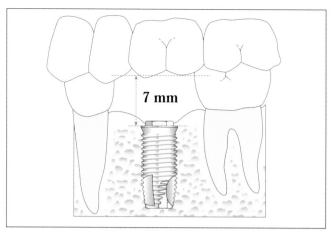

Fig 1-22 Minimal height required for a single-tooth implant (CeraOne abutment).

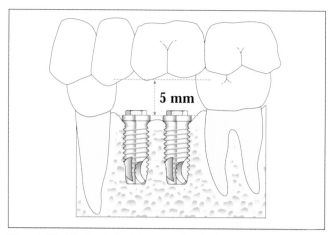

Fig 1-23 Minimal height required for an implant with MirusCone abutment.

■ Height between bone crest and opposing tooth (Figs 1-22 and 1-23)
The vertical height between the bone crest and the opposing tooth defines the maximum height of the implant reconstruction. With a single-tooth abutment, such as CeraOne, a minimum of 6.5 mm is required. However a minimum of 7 mm should be planned. With a MirusCone abutment, it is possible to realize a reconstruction with a minimum height of 5 mm.

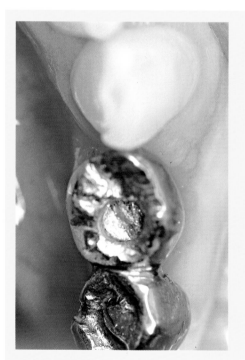

NOTE
With an available height of 5 mm, the gold screws cannot be covered by resin composite.

Fig 1-24 Occlusal view of an implant-supported prosthetic restoration. Because of the small available interarch height, and despite the use of a MirusCone abutment, it is not possible to cover the heads of the prosthetic gold screws. The screw heads may be damaged over time and become difficult to loosen if a complication arises.

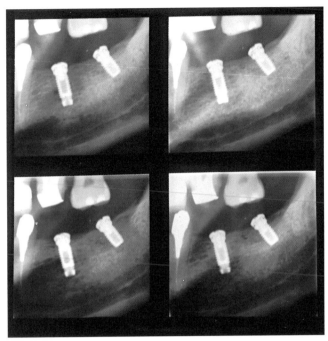

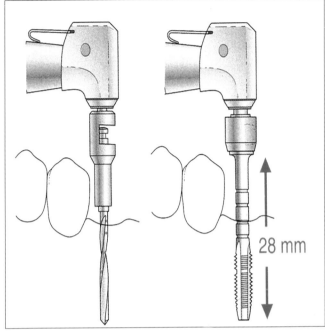

Fig 1-25 Radiographic evaluation 3 months after placement of two implants in the mandibular left segment. Despite the available bone volume, it was possible to place only a 7-mm implant distally, and with a mesial orientation. This is due to the uncompensated encroachment of the maxillary second molar, which has obstructed the passage of surgical instruments. It is important to always verify the free access to the implant site, even in patients with normal jaw opening. The encroachment should be eliminated before the surgical phase. (Radiography by Dr G. Pasquet and Dr R. Cavezian.)

Fig 1-26 Obstruction is inherently associated with drill extensions. Sometimes the large height of an adjacent crown requires use of a drill extension in the posterior segments. However, in these regions, the interarch height usually does not permit passage of the extension, and the implant placement might be compromised.

■ Interarch distance at maximal opening (Figs 1-25 and 1-26)

Access to the implant site should be evaluated even if the patient has an acceptable oral opening. If an overerupted opposing tooth is not compensated for, it could interfere with the instruments or restrict the free passage of instruments or screwdrivers. The occlusal curve should be corrected before implant placement.

■ Mesiodistal distance

With Regular Platform implants, a mesiodistal distance of 7 mm, center to center, is necessary for avoiding interference between implants or implant and teeth. For Narrow Platform, 6 mm is required, and for Wide Platform 8 mm is the minimum distance. In situations where several implants are to be placed, these numbers have to be multiplied to determine the total distance.

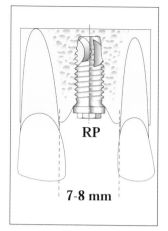

Fig 1-27 Minimum mesiodistal space required for treating a single-tooth loss with a Regular Platform (RP) implant.

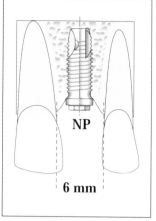

Fig 1-28 Minimum mesiodistal space required for treating a single-tooth loss with a Narrow Platform (NP) implant.

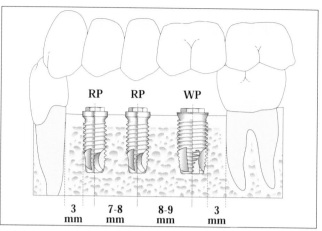

Fig 1-29 Minimum mesiodistal space required for treating partial edentulism with Regular Platform (RP) and Wide Platform (WP) implants.

Functional evaluation

The functional checklist includes control of abrasion facets, significant tooth wear, parafunction, and so on. The greater the functional risk of a patient, the more important it is that the number of implants equal the number of roots replaced. The number of implants, their diameters, and their positions are determined by the biomechanical demands of each edentulous situation. The radiographic evaluation must confirm the suggested implant solution. If not, the implant solution should be avoided.

Classification of functional risks
Favorable occlusal context
Balanced occlusion
No temporomandibular joint pathosis
Regular excursive movement of the mandible
Moderately unfavorable occlusal context
Presence of small wear facets
Development of high masticatory forces
Unfavorable occlusal condition without parafunction (eg, Class II, division 2, occlusion)
Reduced interarch height
Highly unfavorable occlusal context
Bruxism
Parafunction
Posterior bite collapse
Presence of large wear facets
History of cracks or fractures of natural teeth
History of repeated cracks or fractures of prostheses or veneers

Radiographic examination *(Figs 1-30 to 1-35)*

For the first consultations, the retroalveolar or panoramic radiographic examination is sufficient for evaluating the possibility of implant placement.

The examination of these radiographs is used:

- To verify the feasibility of implant placement by evaluation of the bone height, especially over the inferior alveolar nerve and under the sinus cavity. If the height appears to be sufficient, a computerized tomographic scan or a Scanora should be prescribed.
- To determine any risks related to vertical bone resorption
- To look for bone pathoses:
  - All acute infections must be treated before implant placement.
  - Chronic lesions (periapical granuloma, etc) close to the implant zone must be treated and healed before implant placement.
  - Chronic lesions (periapical granuloma, etc) distant from the implant zone (in the opposing arch or contralateral sector) can be treated after implant placement, provided that the implants are subgingival.
- To evaluate periodontal status.

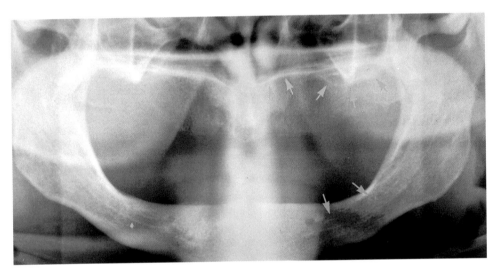

Fig 1-30 Panoramic radiograph of a patient who is completely edentulous in both arches. This examination is sufficient for evaluating if implant treatment is possible. The anatomic structures are easily recognized: inferior alveolar nerve (blue arrow), maxillary sinus (red arrow), and nasal cavities (green arrow). However, this investigation does not allow an evaluation of the available bone volume. (Radiography by Dr G. Pasquet and Dr R. Cavezian.)

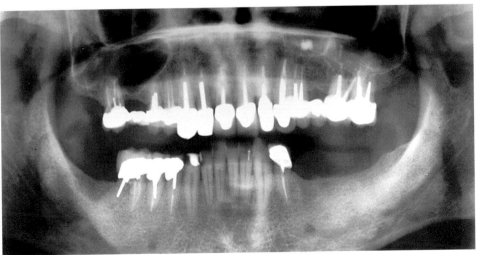

Fig 1-31 A panoramic radiograph of a patient who is edentulous in the mandibular left segment indicates that the height of the available bone over the alveolar nerve may be sufficient for implant placement. A computerized tomographic scan or Scanora should be prescribed.

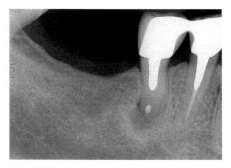 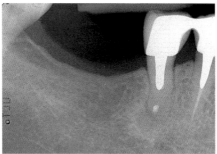 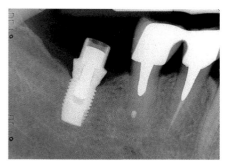

Fig 1-32 A retroalveolar radiograph of the mandibular right segment indicates that implant treatment may be a good solution. Note the signs of inflammation at the apex of the first premolar. Apical surgery has been performed and a retrograde filling placed.

Fig 1-33 Same patient. Six months after apical surgery, the lesion has practically disappeared. Implants can be placed.

Fig 1-34 Same patient. Radiographic evaluation 3 months after implant placement.

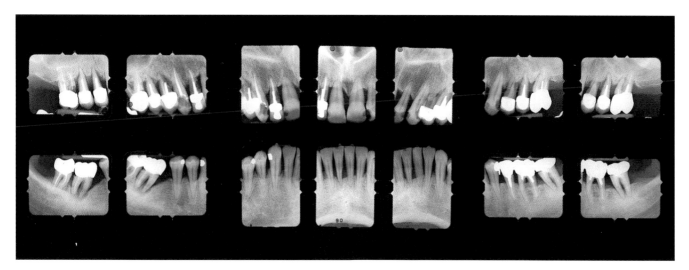

Fig 1-35 A retroalveolar overview could be used for the preliminary examination; however, a three-dimensional bone assessment is necessary for the final implant treatment planning.

Periodontal control

Although the periodontal examination is the last one on this list, it represents an inevitable step in the preimplant evaluation. A number of studies have shown that the peri-implant tissues are susceptible to infections caused by pathogenic bacteria originating from the periodontal pockets around natural teeth. It is, therefore, important to ensure the good health of the periodontal tissues before implant placement is commenced.

A peri-implant treatment protocol is often necessary to improve the quality of the tissue around the implant abutment.

It is possible to place the implants after the initial preparation phase and to use the subgingival implant period to undertake periodontal treatment in the dentate segment.

Suggested Readings

Clinical preimplant examination

Assémat-Tessandier X, Amzalag G. La décision en implantologie. Paris, CDP, 1993.

Renouard F. Examen clinique pré implantaire. Critèares de choix. Act Odontostomatol 1996;5:345-357.

Natural tooth or dental implant?

Lewis S. Treatment planning: Teeth versus implants. Int J Periodont Rest Dent 1996;16:367-377.

Tobacco and implants

Bain CA. Smoking and implant failure: Benefits of a smoking cessation protocol. Int J Oral Maxillofac Implants 1996;11:756-759.

Bain CA, Moy PK. The association between the failure of dental implants and cigarette smoking. Int J Oral Maxillofac Implants 1993;8:609-615.

De Bruyn H, Collaert B. The effect of smoking on early failure. Clin Oral Implants Res 1994;5:260-264.

Inflammation of peri-implant tissue

Beglundh T, Lindhe J, Ericsson I, Marinello CP, Liljenborg B, Thompsen P. The soft tissue barrier at implants and teeth. Clin Oral Implants Res 1991;2:81-90.

Brägger U, Bürgin WB, Hämmerle CHF, Lang NP. Association between clinical parameters assessed around implants and teeth. Clin Oral Implants Res 1997;8:412-421.

Gouvoussis J, Doungkamol S, Yeung S. Cross-infection from periodontitis sites to failing implant sites in the same mouth. Int J Oral Maxillofac Implants 1997;12:666-673.

Quirynen M, Listgarten MA. The distribution of bacterial morphotypes around natural teeth and titanium implants ad modum Brånemark. Clin Oral Implants Res 1990;1:8-12.

Osteoporosis and implants

Dao TTT, Anderson D, Zarb GA. Is osteoporosis a risk factor for osseointegration of dental implants? Int J Oral Maxillofac Implants 1993;8:137-143.

Implant risk patients

Etienne D, Sanz M, Aroca S, Barbieri B, Ohayoun JP. Identification of risk patients in oral implantology. Part 2. J Parodontol Implant Orale 1998;3:273-297.

Roche Y. Chirurgie dentaire et patients à risque. Evaluation et précautions à pendre en pratique quotidienne. Paris: Flammarion, 1996.

Sanz M, Etienne D. Identification of risk patients in oral implantology. Part 1. J Parodontol Implant Orale 1998;3:257-272.

Smith RA, Berger R, Dodson TB. Risk factors associated with dental implants in healthy and medically compromised patients. Int J Oral Maxillofac Implants 1992;7:367-372.

Irradiation and implants

Franzén L, Rosenquist JB, Rosenquist KI, Gustafsson I. Oral implant rehabilitation of patients with oral malignancies treated with radiotherapy and surgery without adjunctive hyperbaric oxygen. Int J Oral Maxillofac Implants 1997;10:183-187.

Ueda M, Kaneda T, Takahashi H. Effect of hyperbaric oxygen therapy on osseointegration of titanium implants in irradiated bone: A preliminary report. Int J Oral Maxillofac Implants 1993;8:41-44.

Implants and adolescents

Brugnolo E, Mazzano C, Cordioli G, Majzoub Z. Clinical and radiographic findings following placement of single-tooth implants in young patients. Case reports. Int J Periodont Rest Dent 1996;16:421-433.

Koch G, Bergendal T, Kvint S, Johansson UB. Consensus Conference on Oral Implants in Young Patients. Jönköping, Sweden, The Institute for Postgraduate Dental Education, 1996.

Additional readings

Nevins M, Mellonig JT. Implant Therapy: Clinical Approaches and Evidence of Success, vol 2. Chicago: Quintessence, 1998.

Zitzmann NU, Schärer P. Ein klinisches Kompendium. Zurich, Kolb, 1997.

Chapter 2

Esthetic Risk Factors

After having been seen for a long time as merely a functional screw-retained prosthesis, implant prosthetics have found a major indication in restoration of anterior edentulous areas. All the components necessary for offering the patient the best of esthetic results exist today.

However, even if scrupulous respect has been paid to the surgical and prosthetic protocols, the result is not always satisfactory. This is related to the fact that there are certain specific parameters that must be considered for the esthetic implant-supported prosthesis. Therefore, a specific clinical examination is necessary to investigate and evaluate esthetic risk factors.

There are several types of esthetic risk factors:

- Gingival risk factors
- Dental risk factors
- Bone risk factors
- Patient risk factors

	Okay	Caution
Gingival risk factors		
Smile line	Dental	Gingival
Gingiva	Thick and fibrous	Fine
Thickness of keratinized gingiva	≥5 mm	<2 mm
Papillae of adjacent teeth	Flat	Scalloped
Dental risk factors		
Form of natural teeth	Squared	Triangular
Interdental contact	Surface	Point
Position of interdental contact	<5 mm above the bone	>5 mm above the bone
Bone risk factors		
Vestibular concavity	Absent	Present
Adjacent implants	No	Yes
Vertical bone resorption	No	Yes
Proximal bony peaks	Yes	No
Patient risk factors		
Esthetic requirements		High
Hygiene level and availability	Good	Poor
Provisionalization	Stable	Unstable

Gingival Risk Factors

Smile line *(Figs 2-1 and 2-2)*

The smile line is the first parameter to evaluate for restorations in the esthetic sectors. A gingival smile could represent a relative contraindication, especially if other risk factors are associated. In that case, a traditional prosthetic solution should be considered. If the implant solution is selected, the patient must be informed about the difficulties and the esthetic risk associated with the treatment.

Gingival quality *(Figs 2-3 and 2-4)*

The thicker and more fibrous the gingiva, the better the esthetic result. Too-thin gingiva is more difficult to manipulate and does not always mask the implant and abutment metal parts.

A good height of the keratinized gingiva is also necessary, not only for the tissue health around the implant but also for an improved esthetic result.

Papillae of adjacent teeth *(Figs 2-5 and 2-6)*

The papillary morphology of the adjacent natural teeth is an important parameter to consider. If the papillae are long and fine, it is difficult to obtain a perfect esthetic result. On the other hand, if the papillae are thick and short, their "natural regeneration" is facilitated.

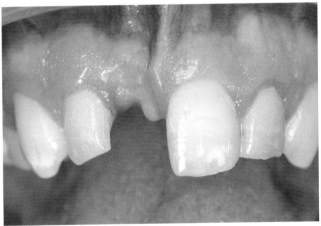

Fig 2-1 The maxillary right central incisor has been lost to trauma. A partial denture has replaced the lost tooth provisionally. The loss of tissue necessitates bone regeneration or bone grafting.

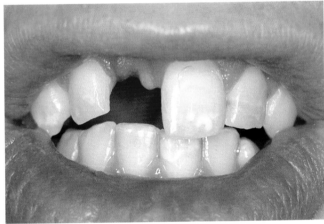

Fig 2-2 Same patient. The smile shows gingiva, and the situation is associated with a considerable esthetic risk factor.

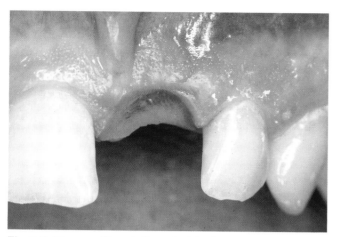

Fig 2-3 The maxillary left central incisor has been lost to trauma. Note the quality and thickness of the keratinized mucosa. This situation is favorable for an implant-supported prosthesis.

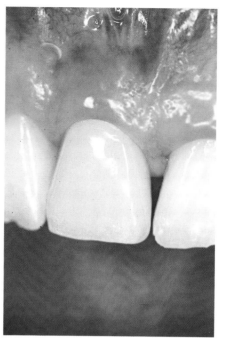

Fig 2-4 An implant-supported prosthesis has replaced the maxillary right central incisor. Note the thin peri-implant mucosa. The esthetic result is not satisfactory.

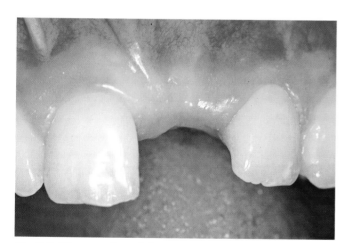

Fig 2-5 The maxillary left central incisor has been lost to trauma. The interdental papillae of the adjacent natural teeth are thick and short. The prognosis for their regeneration around the implant prosthesis is good. (The final result is presented in Fig 2-7.)

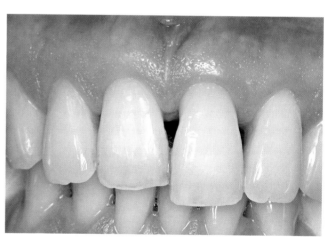

Fig 2-6 The maxillary left central incisor is to be replaced with an implant-supported prosthesis. Note the winding of the gingiva. Complete regeneration of the papillae around the implants will be difficult to achieve.

Dental Risk Factors

Form of natural teeth *(Figs 2-7 and 2-8)*

The more square the tooth forms, the easier it is to achieve good esthetics. Triangular tooth forms represent a risk factor, especially because the need for papillary regeneration is greater in these situations and the implant positioning has to be more precise.

Position of interdental point of contact

If the interdental contact is found less than 5 mm from the bone margin, papillary regeneration takes place in practically all cases. If the position is more than 5 mm from the bone margin, the chance of papillary regeneration decreases as the distance between the point and the marginal bone increases.

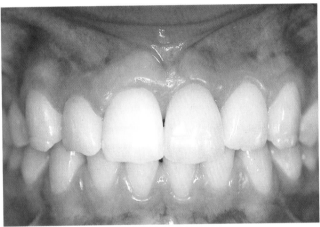

Fig 2-7 The maxillary left central incisor has been replaced with an implant prosthesis (see Fig 2-5). The square form of the teeth represents a favorable situation for the regeneration of the interdental papillae. (Prosthesis by Dr D. Vilbert and S. Tissier.)

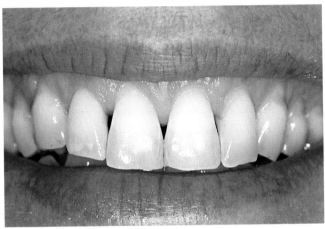

Fig 2-8 The maxillary right first premolar should be replaced with an implant prosthesis. Note the triangular form of the teeth and the lack of papillae filling the interdental space. This situation should be considered to represent an esthetic risk, especially because the patient's smile reveals a large gingival area.

Shape of the interdental contact

The larger the interdental contact surface, the smaller the papillary space and the simpler the papillary regeneration.

Bone Risk Factors

Vestibular concavity *(Figs 2-9 to 2-11)*

The presence of a vestibular concavity represents an important esthetic risk factor. Bone regeneration or grafting is needed before the implant is placed, or the implant will have to be placed following the bone crest, but with an unfavorable orientation of the prosthesis axis.

Adjacent implants *(Figs 2-12 to 2-14)*

Even if papillary regeneration occurs naturally at a natural tooth, it is difficult to achieve between two implants because of the absence of a bony papilla (septum) in that situation.

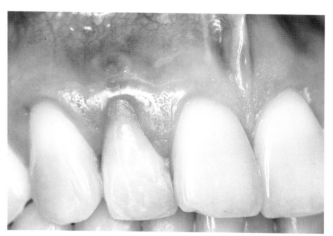

Fig 2-10 Same patient. The gingival level seems appropriate for an esthetic restoration.

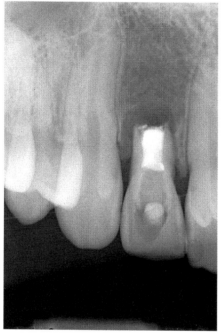

Fig 2-9 A retroalveolar radiograph reveals a significant resorption of the maxillary right lateral incisor. An implant tooth replacement is planned.

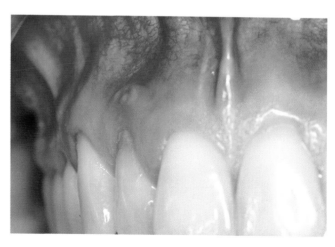

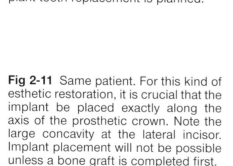

Fig 2-11 Same patient. For this kind of esthetic restoration, it is crucial that the implant be placed exactly along the axis of the prosthetic crown. Note the large concavity at the lateral incisor. Implant placement will not be possible unless a bone graft is completed first.

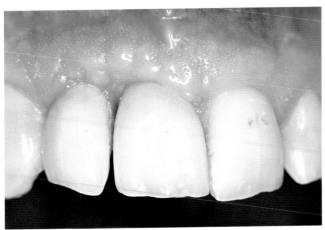

Fig 2-12 The maxillary right central and lateral incisors have been replaced with single-tooth implants (CeraOne abutment). Note the absence of papilla between the implants at the follow-up 3 years after implant loading. (Prostheses by Dr J. Bunni and J.-J. Sansemat.)

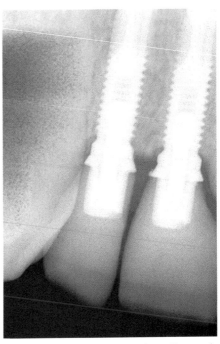

Fig 2-13 Same patient. A radiograph at the follow-up examination 3 years after loading reveals the proximity of the implants and the absence of peaks of bony septae between the implants, explaining the lack of gingival papillae. The use of a Narrow Platform implant with STR abutment in the position of the lateral incisor would certainly have improved the result.

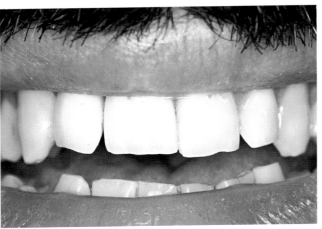

Fig 2-14 Same patient smiling. His smile does not reveal much of the gingiva.

Vertical bone resorption *(Figs 2-15 to 2-17)*

Vertical bone resorption, resulting from trauma or periodontal disease, leads to a difference between the bone level where the implants are to be placed and the bone level of the adjacent teeth. If the implant is placed much deeper (more than 3 mm) than the line connecting the approximating cementoenamel junctions, the prosthetic crown may not be aligned with the adjacent teeth.

Proximal bony peaks *(Fig 2-18)*

The retroalveolar radiograph will reveal the presence or absence of bony septa proximal to adjacent teeth. It is on these peaks that the gingival papillae can be formed.

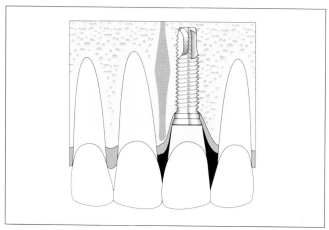

Fig 2-15 The risks associated with placing the implant too far apically.

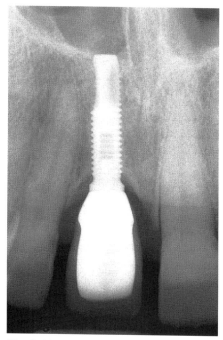

Fig 2-16 A retroalveolar radiograph of an implant restoration 3 years after loading reveals peri-implant bone stability. Note the deep countersinking of the implant relative to the line connecting the approximating cementoenamel junctions.

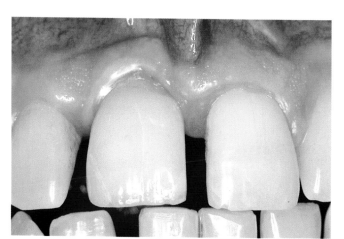

Fig 2-17 Same patient. There is a lack of harmony between the natural teeth and the implant crowns. Completion of bone grafting or bone regeneration procedures before implant placement would have eliminated the problem.

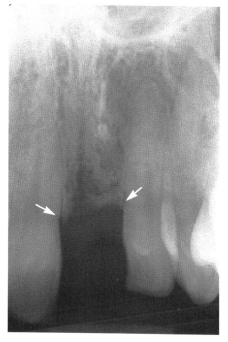

Fig 2-18 Preoperative retroalveolar radiograph of the area of the maxillary left central incisor, which has been lost to trauma. The radiograph shows the absence of peaks of bony saptae proximally *(arrows)*. Papillary regeneration will be more difficult.

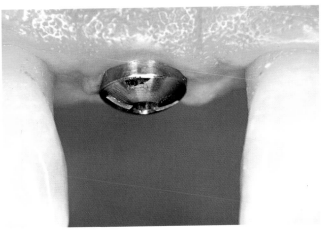

Fig 2-19 A single-tooth implant has been used to replace the maxillary right central incisor. The patient had periodontal disease, which was treated before implant surgery. Note the health and quality of the tissues around the healing abutment.

Patient Risk Factors

Esthetic requirements

It is very important to identify patients who have unrealistic esthetic demands. The higher the esthetic requirements, the more cooperative the patient should be and the more important it is that he or she be aware of the difficulties, the limitations, and the duration of the treatment.

Hygiene level *(Figs 2-19 to 2-21)*

Extremely rigorous dental hygiene and good plaque control must be exercised by the patient to obtain the expected esthetic results. If not, the presence of permanent inflammation, even minor, may compromise the quality and healing capacity of the gingiva.

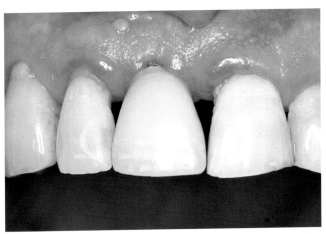

Fig 2-20 Same patient at the 2-year follow-up. Note the inflammation of the soft tissue (gingivitis and mucositis) and the presence of bacterial plaque. Mucosal recession is visible at the crown-implant interface. The CeraOne abutment will become visible.

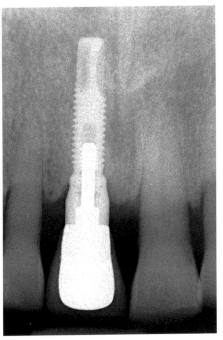

Fig 2-21 Same patient. Radiograph at the 2-year follow-up.

Provisionalization *(Figs 2-22 to 2-24)*

The provisional restoration should be stable and not compromise the patient's ability to perform plaque control. If a denture is used, it should be designed to avoid all movements that interfere with the implant zone. A metal structure represents a good option for this type of provisional restoration.

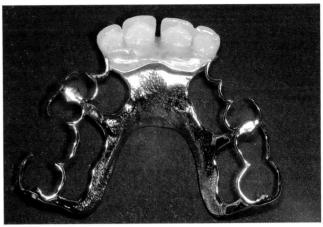

Fig 2-22 A partial denture is the simplest solution for securing provisional restoration during the implant-healing phase. However, its instability may cause severe mucosal problems. In situations aiming for an esthetic restoration, a denture with a metal framework might be considered.

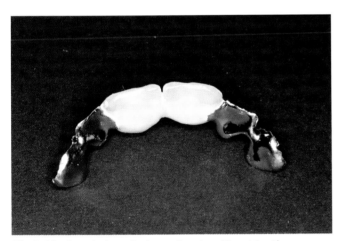

Fig 2-23 A resin-bonded prosthesis without tooth preparation represents an ideal solution for provisional restoration in situations aiming for an esthetic result. However, their cost and the problem of their bond strength make this solution difficult to use.

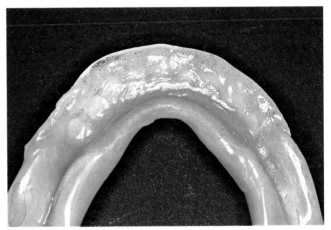

Fig 2-24 The completely edentulous arch represents a certain risk because of the difficulty in obtaining a stable and atraumatic solution for provisionalization. It is important to follow such patients very regularly for early detection of any trauma to the mucosa. The denture base (especially at the anterior sector) should be remade, at a minimum, every month.

Suggested readings

Arnoux JP, Weisgold AS, Lu J. Single-tooth anterior implant: A word of caution. Part I. J Esthet Dent 1997;9:225-233.

Jemt T. Regeneration of gingival papilla after single-implant treatment. Int J Periodont Rest Dent 1997;17:327-333.

Salama H, Salama M, Garber D, Adar P. Developing optimal peri-implant papillae within the esthetic zone: Guided soft tissue augmentation. J Esthet Dent 1995;7:125-129.

Tarnow DP, Magner AW, Fletcher P. The effect of the distance from the contact point to the crest of bone on the presence or absence of the interproximal dental papilla. J Periodontol 1992;63:995-996.

Weisgold AS, Arnoux JP, Lu J. Single-tooth anterior implant: A word of caution. Part II. J Esthet Dent 1997:9:285-294.

Additional reading

Palacci P, Ericsson I, Engstrand P, Rangert B. Optimal Implant Positioning and Soft Tissue Management for the Brånemark System. Chicago: Quintessence, 1995.

Chapter 3

Biomechanical Risk Factors

A good understanding of implant biomechanics makes it possible to optimize the treatment plan for each patient to reduce the risk of functional complications and failures.

The presence of one risk factor is not necessarily a contraindication to implant treatment. On the other hand, the presence of several risk factors represents a risky situation. For example, the use of two implants to support a three-unit prosthesis in the posterior region for a patient who exhibits bruxism, with the implant offset from the center of the prosthetic crown, represents a major risk.

A retrospective analysis has been done to identify and evaluate risk factors based on the study of a large number of complications and failures. This evaluation in not strictly scientifically valid but nevertheless allows a ranking of different biomechanical risk factors.

During the treatment-planning process, it is possible to identify and evaluate different risk factors with support from the tables in this chapter.

A score is assigned to each risk factor. The sum of these values represents the Biomechanical Risk Score for the specific clinical situation. If the score is less than 2.0, no particular risk is foreseen. A score of 2.0 to 3.0 represents a moderate to major risk, while a score higher than 3.0 indicates a contraindication for the implant treatment plan envisioned. It is, however, always possible to modify the treatment plan by adding an extra implant or adjusting the prosthesis or occlusal scheme, for example.

If a complication occurs after treatment, it is a good idea to review the biomechanical checklist and adjust the treatment accordingly, to eliminate the cause of the problem.

	Okay	Caution	Danger
Biomechanical risk score	<2.0	2.0–3.0	>3.0

Note: The score value for each risk situation is based on an "average" clinical situation. These values may be adjusted, depending on the specific clinical situation. For example, the presence of a lateral incisor extension may represent the value 0.5, while a molar extension represents a value of 1.0.

Several types of biomechanical risk factors may be defined:

- *Geometric risk factors:* number of implants, their relative position, and prosthesis geometry
- *Occlusal risk factors:* significant lateral contact in excursive jaw movements and parafunctional habits
- *Bone and implant risk factors:* dependence on newly formed bone in the absence of good initial mechanical stability and implant diameter that is considerably smaller than the ideal for the situation.
- *Technological risk factors:* lack of prosthetic fit and cemented prostheses.

- *Alarm signals:* indication of overload during clinical function

Note

The presence of several factors indicates a risky situation for the implants and prosthesis.

Geometric Risk Factors

Geometric risk	Score
Number of implants (N) less than number of root supports (for N<3)	1
Use of Wide Platform implants (per implant)	−1
Implant connected to a natural tooth	0.5
Implants placed in tripod configuration	−1
Presence of a prosthetic extension (per pontic)	1
Implants placed offset from the center of the prosthesis	1
Excessive height of the restoration	0.5

Number of implants less than number of root supports *(Fig 3-1)*

To define the ideal number of implants in a given clinical situation, it is not sufficient to consider the number of teeth. It is necessary to consider the number of root supports to replace. For example, a canine represents one root support, while a molar represents two root supports.

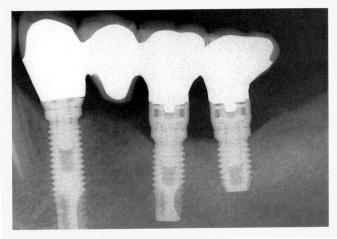

Note

This evaluation is especially important for restorations supported by fewer than three implants. For restorations based on three implants or more, it is possible to use fewer implants than root supports without substantial increase in load (Fig 3-1).

Fig 3-1 Radiograph at follow-up 4 years after loading. Note the marginal bone stability, achieved despite the use of short implants. Even if this situation reveals reduced support (three implants for five roots), no substantial load increase is foreseen due to the inherent stability offered by the splinting of the three implants.

One implant replacing a molar (Figs 3-2 to 3-6)

A molar needs to be supported by two or three roots to avoid the crown to extend over the roots. Use of one Regular Platform implant for a molar restoration, therefore, generates a geometric risk score of 2.0 (number of implants less than number of root supports plus a prosthetic extension). The risk score may be reduced by using one Wide Platform (–1.0) or two Regular Platform implants.

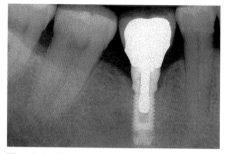

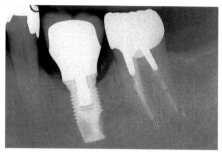

Fig 3-2 Radiograph at the 4-year follow-up. The mandibular right first molar has been replaced by an implant-supported prosthesis. Note the large difference between the implant diameter and the mesiodistal width of the crown. This situation should be considered to represent a biomechanical risk. (Prosthesis by Dr P. Simonet and A. Pinault.)

Fig 3-3 Radiograph at the 1-year follow-up. The mandibular left first molar has been replaced by an implant-supported prosthesis. The use of a Wide Platform implant provides a favorable biomechanical situation. (Prosthesis by Dr P. Simonet and A. Lecardonnel.)

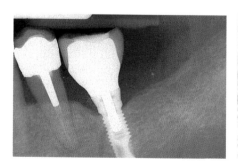

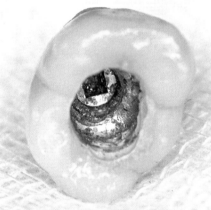

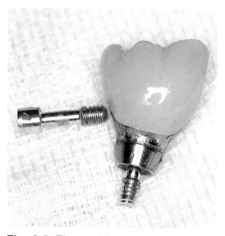

Fig 3-4 Radiograph at follow-up. A Regular Platform implant has replaced the mandibular right first molar. Note the large height of the crown, its mesiodistal width relative to the implant diameter, and the fact that the implant is the distal support in the arch.

Fig 3-5 Same patient. The gold screw of the CeraOne abutment has loosened and the crown has become mobile. In this situation, it is difficult to break the crown cement from the abutment without damaging the internal thread of the implant. One solution is to pierce the crown and retighten the gold screw. *Note: For cemented restorations, it is suggested that the access to the abutment screw be marked with a slightly different color of ceramic.*

Fig 3-6 The gold screw had to be changed. However, if the prosthetic concept is not modified, there is a risk that the complication will reoccur. Also, if the fixture has a diameter smaller than 4 mm, it will be at risk of fracturing.

Two implants supporting three roots or more *(Figs 3-7 to 3-9)*

Replacing three or more root supports with two Regular Platform implants results in a geometric risk score of 1.0 (number of implants less than number of root supports). If two Wide Platform implants are used, this risk factor is eliminated.

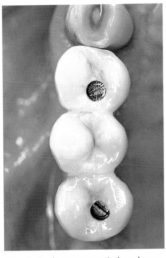

Fig 3-7 A screw-retained provisional prosthesis is fastened to the implants in a patient who exhibits bruxism. Two Regular Platform implants (one in position 14 and one mesially to position 16) replace three teeth. This situation should be considered to be associated with a certain risk. (Prosthesis by Dr J.-M. Gonzalez, Dr P. Rajzbaum, and C. Laval.)

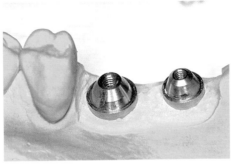

Fig 3-8 Working cast during the construction of a prosthesis to replace the mandibular left first and second molars. Note the use of a Wide Platform implant in position 36 and a Regular Platform, 4-mm diameter, implant in position 37. This situation is favorable.

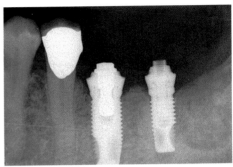

Fig 3-9 Same patient. Radiograph taken at the placement of the final abutments.

Use of Wide Platform implants *(Fig 3-10)*

The Wide Platform implant provides increased mechanical strength and greater load support than a Regular Platform implant.

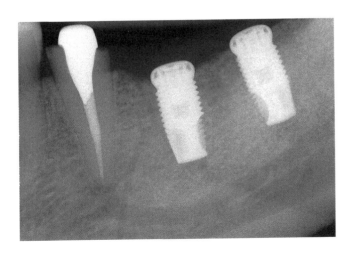

Note

The use of a wide implant in situations of very dense bone may lead to marginal bone resorption during the healing period. Therefore, use of this implant in Type I bone is not recommended.

Fig 3-10 Radiograph taken before second-stage surgery. When bone volume and density allow, the use of Wide Platform implants offers an improved biomechanical resistance.

Implant connected to natural teeth *(Figs 3-11 to 3-14)*

Combining two systems with a great difference in rigidity (teeth have a mobility on the order of 10 times greater than that of implants) may result in unbalanced load sharing between the supports. This situation is assigned a geometric risk factor of 0.5. However, this factor is often combined with other geometric factors, such as lack of bone support and extension (see Fig 3-32).

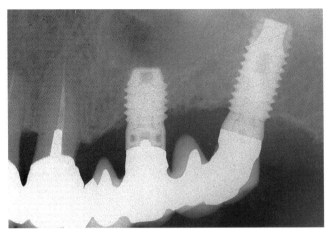

Fig 3-11 Retroalveolar radiograph. Two Wide Platform implants have been placed in the maxillary left quadrant. Their positions have been determined by available bone volume. A connection to natural teeth has been made. This situation should be considered to be associated with a certain risk.

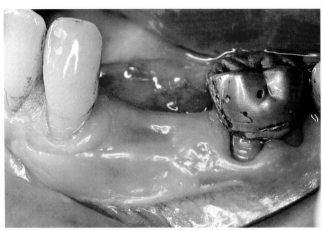

Fig 3-12 Initial clinical view. The mandibular left first and second premolars will be replaced. The mesiodistal distance is not sufficient for placement of two implants under favorable conditions. It was decided to place one implant in position 34 and to connect it to the crown of the first molar.

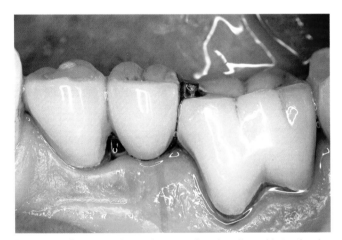

Fig 3-13 Same patient, 1 year after loading. Note the intrusion of the natural tooth. This type of orthodontic movement is associated with the use of connectors that allow vertical movements. If connection is planned, it should be rigid.

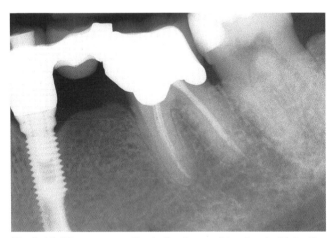

Fig 3-14 The same patient. Radiographic check. Note the gap between the pontic and the natural tooth.

Implants placed in a tripod configuration
(Figs 3-15 and 3-16)

Placement of implants along a straight line at a posterior restoration allows lateral forces to induce adverse bending of the implants. If the implants are placed in a tripod situation, these lateral forces will, to a large extent, be counteracted by more favorable axial forces.

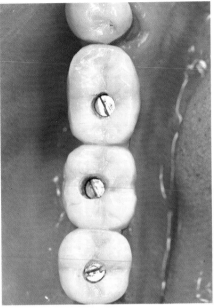
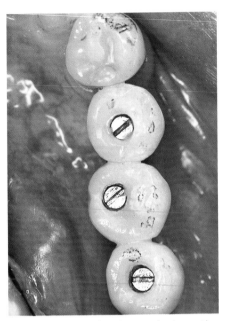

Fig 3-15 Prosthesis replacing the mandibular left second premolar and first and second molars. Note the anteroposterior in-line placement of the implants. This situation does not provide the most effective support for occlusal forces in the lateral direction. (Prosthesis by Dr J.-M. Gonzalez, Dr P. Rajzbaum, and C. Laval.)

Fig 3-16 Prosthesis replacing the mandibular left second premolar and first and second molars. The placement of the implants in a tripod configuration provides better resistance to lateral forces. Note the reduction of the occlusal table widths and the canine guidance for lateral movement. (Prosthesis by Dr G. Tirlet and S. Tissier.)

Note

For the complete-arch restoration, in-line placement of implants represents a severe risk of overload. It is important that the implants be spread along the alveolar ridge (Figs 3-17 and 3-18).

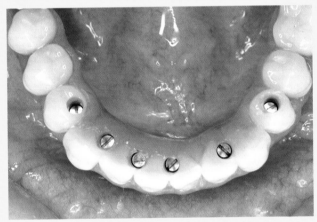
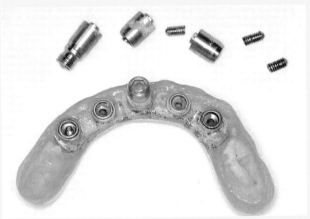

Fig 3-17 For a complete-arch restoration, it is important to spread the implants effectively along the ridge. Note the length of the cantilever extension, which is made possible by the appropriate implant placement.

Fig 3-18 Loosened prosthesis. The placement of the implants in-line, in combination with the large extensions, leads to a risk of mechanical complications, especially if this situation is combined with an unfavorable occlusal context. After several incidences of screw loosening, the abutment screws and two implants fractured.

Presence of a prosthetic extension *(Figs 3-19 and 3-20)*

In any clinical situation, the presence of an extension will considerably increase the load on the implants, and each extension will add 1.0 to the risk score. Generally, a situation with two Regular Platform implants and an extension in the posterior region should not be accepted (geometric risk factor = 2.0), if additional biomechanical risk factors are present.

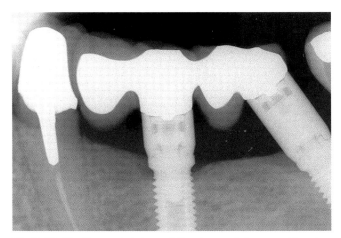

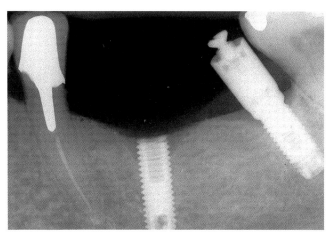

Fig 3-19 Radiograph taken at the 4-year follow-up. Two implants have been used to replace the mandibular left premolars and first molar. Note the anterior extension of the prosthesis.

Fig 3-20 Same patient. The anterior implant is fractured. Several occurrences of screw loosening have preceded this complication.

Implants placed offset from the center of the prosthesis *(Figs 3-21 to 3-24)*

If the implant axis is placed at a distance from the center of the prosthetic crown, there is a risk that the lever arm from the occlusal contact to the implant axis will lead to screw loosening or component fracture. However, if such an offset is a part of a tripod arrangement, it is favorable.

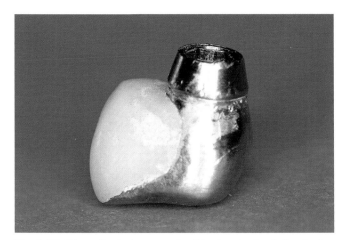

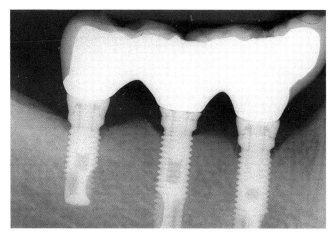

Fig 3-21 The offset placement of the implant relative to the center of the crown is a biomechanical risk factor.

Fig 3-22 Radiograph of an implant-supported prosthesis replacing the mandibular right second premolar and first and second molars.

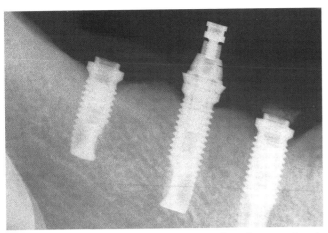

Fig 3-23 Same patient. Six months after the prosthesis was placed, two abutment screws fractured. Several episodes of screw loosening preceded the fractures.

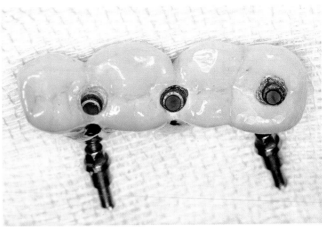

Fig 3-24 Prosthesis and two fractured screws. Note the in-line implant placement and the lingual position of the screw exits. Severe lateral occlusal interference was detected.

Excessive height of the restoration *(Figs 3-25 and 3-26)*

When the height of the abutment-crown complex is substantially increased, the force lever arm to the implant head is increased. If lateral forces arise, there is a risk for screw loosening or component fracture.

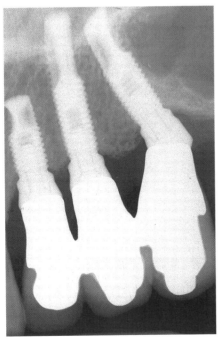

Fig 3-25 Radiograph at the 3-year follow-up. Three implants have been utilized for replacing the maxillary left canine and premolars. The most distal implant is severely inclined to avoid the anterior sinus cavity. Note the large height of the prosthetic crowns.

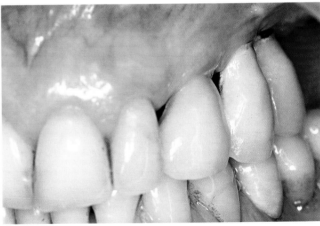

Fig 3-26 Same patient. Note the great height of the prosthetic restoration, as a result of bone resorption. The reduced occlusal tables with low cuspal inclination reduce the lateral forces. This situation, however, should be considered as having a risk.

Occlusal Risk Factors

Occlusal Risk Factors	Score
Bruxism, parafunction, or natural tooth fractures resulting from occlusal factors	2
Lateral occlusal contact on the implant-supported prosthesis only	1
Lateral occlusal contact essentially on adjacent teeth	−1

Bruxism, parafunctional, or natural tooth fractures resulting from occlusal factors *(Fig 3-27)*

The etiology of the tooth loss is a good way to evaluate the occlusal "state" of the patient. Both force intensity and parafunctional habits can have a considerable negative effect on the stability of the implant components. This risk is elevated if the forces are not transmitted through the implant's axis.

A patient who exhibits bruxism or has lost his or her teeth to fracture should be considered a high risk patient, and the implant restoration should be reinforced by optimal support to compensate for the severe loading situation. It is crucial that proper components be used.

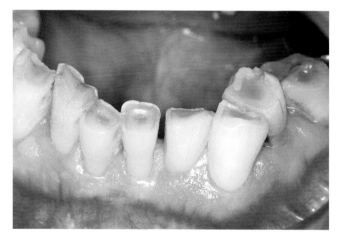

Fig 3-27

Lateral occlusal contact on the implant-supported prostheses only *(Figs 3-28 and 3-29)*

The natural teeth, "suspended" by their periodontal ligament, have a physiologic mobility and a capacity for orthodontic movement. On the contrary, the implants are rigid and fixed in their positions. Therefore, there is a risk that the implants will take a larger charge of the load than the teeth.

To compensate for this risk, the implant prosthesis should ideally be designed in the following way: occlusal contact at the central fossa, low inclination of the cusps, and reduced size of the occlusal table.

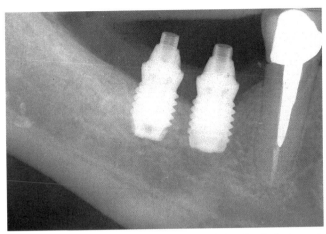

Fig 3-28 Radiograph at placement of the final abutment. Two Regular Platform implants, 5 mm in diameter, have been used to replace the mandibular left first and second molars.

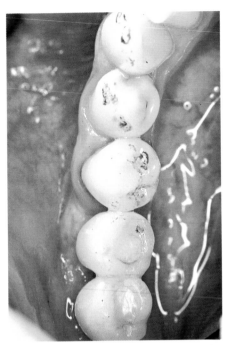

Fig 3-29 Same patient. To limit the lateral forces on the restoration, the occlusal tables have been reduced, and the occlusal scheme is designed so that the natural teeth counteract the lateral forces during excursive movements of the mandible.

Note

Most cases of occlusal overload in the posterior regions are due to lateral forces, which induce bending of the implants. Minimizing or eliminating the lateral contacts will, therefore, significantly reduce the risk of overload (Figs 3-30 and 3-31).

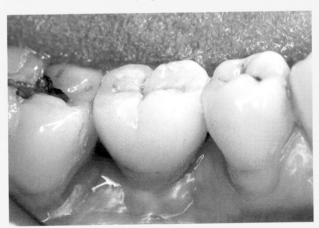

Fig 3-30 Follow-up 3 years after loading. The mandibular right first molar has been replaced with an implant-supported prosthesis. Note the reduced size of the occlusal table.

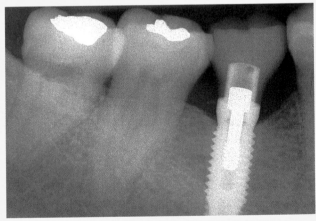

Fig 3-31 Radiograph of the same patient at follow-up 3 years after loading. Note the stable bone level around this Regular Platform, 5-mm-diameter implant. (Prosthesis by Dr J.-C. Bonturi and P. Guillot.)

Note

It is always a good idea to design the prosthesis and position the implants so that the occlusal forces mainly will act along the implant's axes.

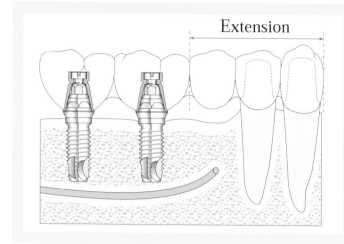

Note

If two or more implants are connected to teeth, the rigidity of the implants makes the implants absorb the major share of the load, and the tooth connection will act more or less as a cantilevered pontic (Fig 3-32). This situation has a high geometric risk score and should be avoided. If performed, lateral contact on the extension should be minimized.

Fig 3-32

Lateral occlusal contact essentially on adjacent teeth *(Figs 3-33 and 3-34)*

Elimination of the lateral contacts on implant-supported prostheses provides a more favorable situation. The proprioceptive capacity of the adjacent teeth may also help to reduce the applied load, particularly during excursive movements of the mandible.

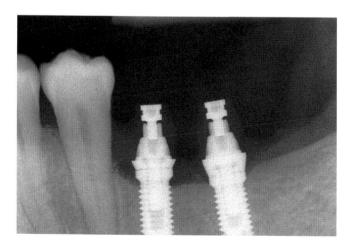

Fig 3-33 Radiograph at placement of the final abutments. The terminal positions of the implants represent a risk.

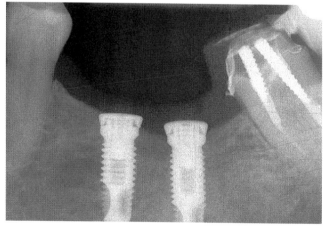

Fig 3-34 Radiograph before second-stage surgery. The mandibular left second molar is going to be restored. The presence of natural teeth distal to the implants represents a favorable situation. The natural teeth may "protect" the implants during function, especially in patients with an unfavorable occlusal context.

Bone and Implant Risk Factors

Bone or implant risk factor	Score
Dependence on newly formed bone in the absence of good initial mechanical stability	1.0
Smaller implant diameter than desired	0.5

After surgery it is important to evaluate the anchorage quality of each implant. It is then possible to define a proper healing time before loading of the prosthesis and to estimate the load capacity of each individual implant.

Dependence on newly formed bone in the absence of good initial mechanical stability

If the primary stability of the implant is not satisfying, the healing time should be extended, and the implant should be protected from too much load during the first period of function. The absence of good primary implant stability should be considered as a risk factor only during the first year of function.

Smaller implant diameter than desired *(Figs 3-35 to 3-37)*

Implants with smaller diameters have a lesser capacity to support bending forces than do implants with larger diameters. In the posterior regions, therefore, a minimum of 4-mm diameter implants should be used. If a Narrow Platform implant is used in the posterior region, this should be considered a major risk factor (+1.0). If a Regular Platform (3.75-mm diameter) implant is used in the posterior region in combination with the stronger gold alloy abutment screw (CeraOne, CerAdapt, TiAdapt), this should be consider a moderate risk factor (+0.5).

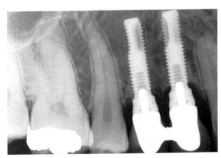

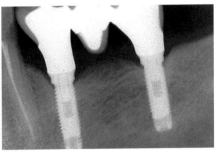

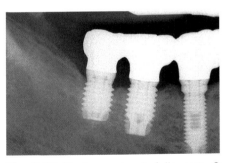

Fig 3-35 Radiograph at follow-up 2 years after loading. A canine and a premolar have been replaced with two 3-mm-diameter implants in this young patient. This situation is associated with a significant risk. The occlusion should be verified regularly for early detection of any overload on the implants. (Prosthesis by Dr P. Simonet and A. Pinault.)

Fig 3-36 Radiograph at follow-up 5 years after loading. The use of two Regular Platform implants to replace three posterior teeth should be considered a risk situation. In this case, the patient has a favorable occlusion, which explains retrospectively the absence of any complications (see the occlusal risk table in chapter 5, page 151). (Prosthesis by Dr M. Jacou and F. Chalard.)

Fig 3-37 Radiograph at follow-up 2 years after loading. The use of 5-mm-diameter Regular Platform implants to replace the molars is ideal, from a biomechanical point of view.

Technological Risk Factors

Technological risk factors	Score
Lack of prosthetic fit or nonoptimal screw joint	0.5
Cemented prostheses	0.5

Lack of prosthetic fit *(Figs 3-38 and 3-39)*

Studies of complete-arch prostheses supported by implants have shown that often there exists misfit between prosthesis and implant. This factor alone does not seem to lead to complications, because there are usually more than enough implants to support the prosthesis. For short-span prostheses in the posterior region, however, where each implant has a strategic value, the lack of prosthetic fit or proper screw tension may become the origin of a complication. Therefore, if precision and screw tightening in the posterior region are not controlled, this should be considered a risk factor.

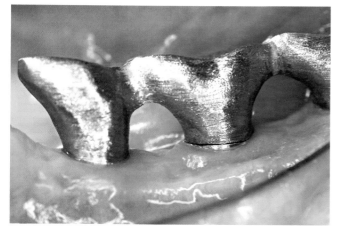 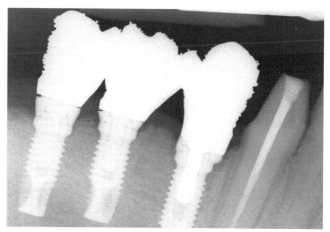

Fig 3-38 Try-in of the metal framework. The gold screws in positions 45 and 47 are tightened. Note the visible gap at position 46, which is due to a vertical misfit.

Fig 3-39 Radiograph at the try-in of a metal framework. Only the anterior gold screw has been tightened. Note the misfit at the two distal implants.

Cemented prostheses *(Figs 3-40 to 3-44)*

If a screw joint will be cemented over, it is important to have a high and stable screw tension, such as is obtained with gold alloy screws (CeraOne, CerAdapt, TiAdapt, or AurAdapt) when a torque controller is used. If this is not the situation, a risk factor is present, because retightening is difficult to accomplish in this situation.

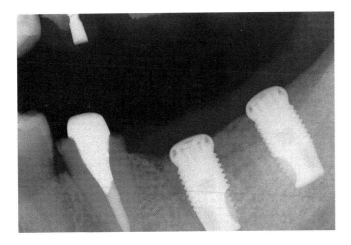

Fig 3-40 Radiograph after healing, showing two implants replacing the mandibular left first and second molars. Two Wide Platform implants have been placed to increase the biomechanical strength of the restoration. The patient does not show any signs of parafunction. The situation is favorable. A cemented-over prosthesis may be chosen.

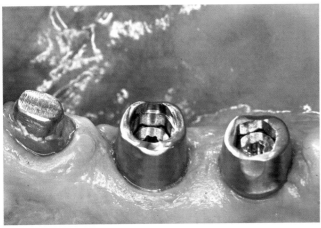

Fig 3-41 Same patient. Two TiAdapt abutments after laboratory preparation. The gold screws are visible.

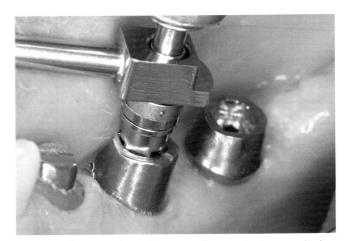

Fig 3-42 Same patient. The use of a countertorque device allows the screws to be tightened to 45 N/cm, which enhances the biomechanical resistance of the system.

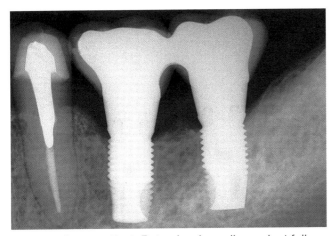

Fig 3-43 Same patient. Retroalveolar radiograph at follow-up 6 months after prosthesis placement.

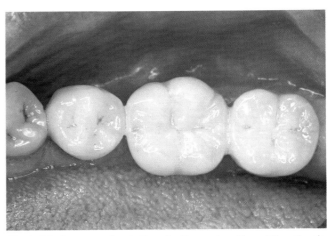

Fig 3-44 Same patient. Prosthetic restoration. (Prosthesis by Dr J.-M. Gonzalez, Dr P. Rajzbaum, and N. Millière.)

Note

It is preferable to use a screw-retained prosthesis in a situation with elevated risk (biomechanical risk score >3). Alarm signals are easier to detect, and complications are easier to handle.

Note

The technological risk factors are often hard to detect in advance. Therefore, to reduce their possible negative influence, the best solution is to use (1) proven and standardized protocols for the prosthesis fabrication, (2) premachined prosthetic components, and (3) tightening instruments with a stable and predefined tightening torque.

Alarm Signals *(Figs 3-45 to 3-51)*

Alarm signals	Score
Repeated loosening of prosthetic or abutment screws	1
Repeated fracture of veneering material (resin or ceramic)	1
Fracture of prosthetic or abutment screws	2
Bone resorption below the first thread of the fixture	1

Brånemark System implants are designed to support prostheses in virtually any clinical situation, provided that the treatment-planning recommendations are followed. However, should overload occur, there are usually signs before the complication leads to failure. Therefore, these alarm signals should not be ignored but rather followed by an analysis of their reason and proper corrective action. In the event of screw loosening or screw fracture, it is not enough to replace and/or retighten the component; the cause of the complication should also be identified and eliminated. If treatment is neglected, the problem may continue and lead to implant failure.

Note

If an alarm signal is found, it is recommended that the aforementioned various biomechanical risk factors be reviewed with the aim of modifying the situation and reducing or eliminating excessive risk factors (for example, by reducing or eliminating cantilevers, modifying the occlusion, inserting extra implants, etc).

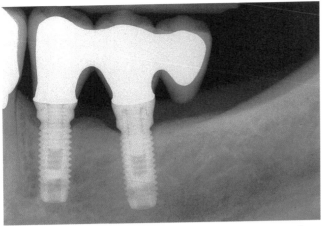

Fig 3-45 Radiograph at follow-up 6 years after loading. Note the distal extension. Note also the stable bone level around the implants. (Prosthesis by Dr T. Meyer and F. Liouville.)

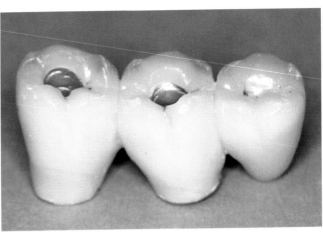

Fig 3-46 Same patient. Prosthesis after removal. The patient asked for a consultation because the prosthesis had loosened. The abutment screw tightness was checked and the gold screws were changed.

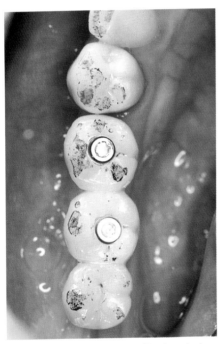

Fig 3-47 Same patient. Occlusal view at maximum intercuspal contact and in lateral excursion. Note the contact at the extension. The occlusion should be modified to suppress the contacts at the prosthetic extensions. If screw loosening occurs a second time, the extension should be eliminated.

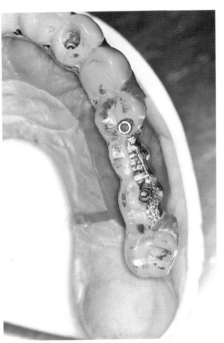

Fig 3-48 Prosthesis on a laboratory cast. Note the fracture on the buccal aspect of the acrylic resin at the second premolar and first molar. This type of complication may be associated with an unfavorable distribution of load or a major occlusal interference. It is essential to find and correct the reason for the problem before the prosthesis is placed in the mouth.

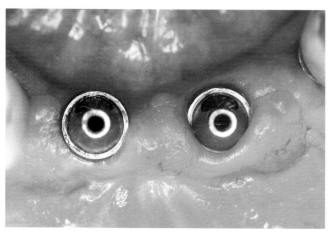

Fig 3-49 Two angulated abutments on implants replacing the mandibular left and right lateral incisors. The extreme lingual orientation of the implants, in combination with an unfavorable occlusal context, has led to screw loosening.

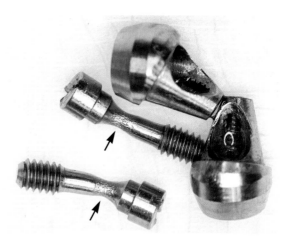

Fig 3-50 Same patient. Note the bending of the abutment screw. Note the deformation zone at the cervical end of the screw *(arrows)*.

Fig 3-51 Radiograph at follow-up 2 years after loading. Two implants have been placed in positions 21 and 23, replacing the maxillary left central and lateral incisors and canine. Note the mesial offset of the central incisor. The patient demonstrates an unfavorable occlusal scheme. The prosthetic gold screws have loosened a number of times. No modification of the prosthetic design has been made. The abutment screw in position 23 eventually fractured. Note the loss of bone at position 23.

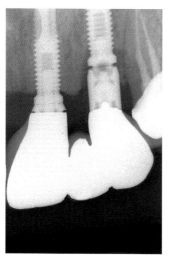

Torque required for optimal tightening of abutment screws*

	Gold	Standard screw	Estheti-Cone	Angulated	Mirus-Cone	CeraOne	CerAdapt	AurAdapt	Ball	TiAdapt
Narrow Platform	10 N/cm	20 N/cm		20 N/cm ideally	20 N/cm	20 N/cm		20 N-cm	20 N/cm	
Regular Platform	10 N/cm	20 N/cm	20 N/cm	20 N/cm ideally	20 N/cm	32 N/cm	32 N/cm	32 N/cm	32 N/cm	20 N/cm
Wide Platform	20 N/cm				32 N/cm	45 N/cm	45 N/cm		45 N/cm	

* Manual tightening mandatory

Clinical Examples Using the Biomechanical Checklist

Case 1 *(Figs 3-52 to 3-55)*

Clinical situation

The patient is edentulous between positions 24 and 26. Three implants have been placed: two Regular Platform, 3.75 mm in diameter; and one Regular Platform, 5 mm in diameter. The restoration is made on EsthetiCone abutments. (Prosthesis by Dr Cardoni and P. Buisson.)

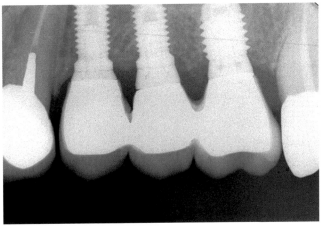

Fig 3-52

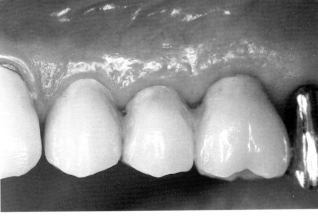

Fig 3-53

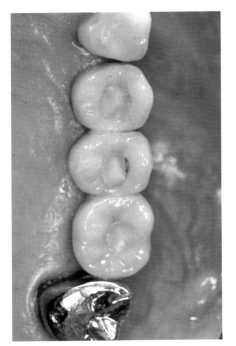

Fig 3-54

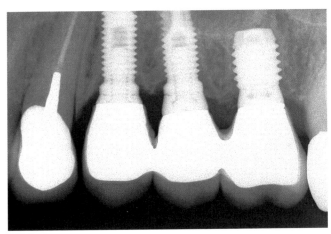

Fig 3-55

Geometric risk factors	Score
Number of implants (N) less than number of root supports (for N<3)	1.0
Use of Wide Platform implants (per implant)	−1.0
Implant connected to a natural tooth	0.5
Implants placed in tripod configuration	−1.0
Presence of a prosthetic extension (per pontic)	1.0
Implants placed offset from the center of the prosthesis	1.0
Excessive height of the restoration	0.5

Occlusal risk factors	Score
Bruxism, parafunction, or natural tooth fractures resulting from occlusal factors	2.0
Lateral occlusal contact on the implant-supported prosthesis only	1.0
Lateral occlusal contact essentially on adjacent teeth	−1.0

Bone and implant risk factors	Score
Dependence on newly formed bone in the absence of good initial mechanical stability	1.0
Smaller implant diameter than desired	0.5

Technological risk factors	Score
Lack of prosthetic fit or nonoptimal screw joint	0.5
Cemented prostheses	0.5

	Okay	Caution	Danger
Biomechanical risk score	<2.0	2.0–3.0	>3.0
Patient's score	−0.5		

Alarm signals	Score
Repeated loosening of prosthetic or abutment screws	1.0
Repeated fracture of veneering material	1.0
Fracture of prosthetic or abutment screws	2.0
Bone resorption below the first thread of the fixture	1.0

Conclusion: excellent functional prognosis, despite the small framework misfit.

Note: The misfit is not visible on the two radiographs because of their projection. This demonstrates the problem of identifying small discrepancies on radiographs.

Case 2 *(Figs 3-56 to 3-59)*

Clinical situation

The patient is edentulous from positions 22 to 26. Two Regular Platform implants have been placed in positions 23 and 25. The restoration is connected to the natural tooth in position 27. The patient does not show any signs of bruxism or parafunction. (Prosthesis by Dr F. Decup and S. Tissier.)

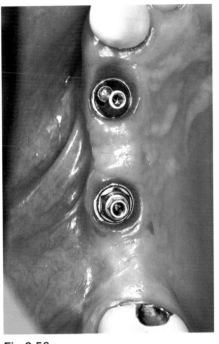

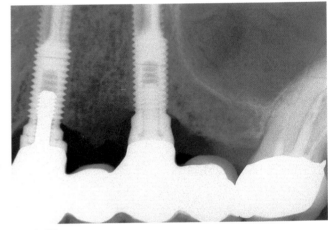

Fig 3-56

Fig 3-57

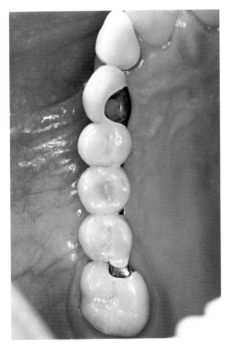

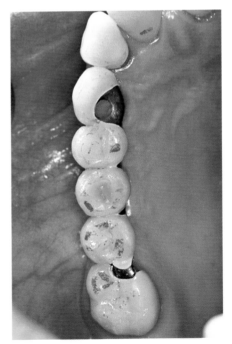

Fig 3-58

Fig 3-59

Geometric risk factors	Score
Number of implants (N) less than number of root supports (for N<3)	1.0
Use of Wide Platform implants (per implant)	−1.0
Implant connected to a natural tooth	0.5
Implants placed in tripod configuration	−1.0
Presence of a prosthetic extension (per pontic)	1.0
Implants placed offset from the center of the prosthesis	1.0
Excessive height of the restoration	0.5

Occlusal risk factors	Score
Bruxism, parafunction, or natural tooth fractures resulting from occlusal factors	2.0
Lateral occlusal contact on the implant-supported prosthesis only	1.0
Lateral occlusal contact essentially on adjacent teeth	−1.0

Bone and implant risk factors	Score
Dependence on newly formed bone in the absence of good initial mechanical stability	1.0
Smaller implant diameter than desired	0.5

Technological risk factors	Score
Lack of prosthetic fit or nonoptimal screw joint	0.5
Cemented prostheses	0.5

	Okay	Caution	Danger
Biomechanical risk score	<2.0	2.0–3.0	>3.0
Patient's score		2.0	

Alarm signals	Score
Repeated loosening of prosthetic or abutment screws	1.0
Repeated fracture of veneering material (resin or ceramic)	1.0
Fracture of prosthetic or abutment screws	2.0
Bone resorption below the first thread of the fixture	1.0

Conclusion: The patient demonstrates a moderate functional risk (3.0) and at any alarm signal the prosthesis design should be modified. One solution is to place an extra implant.

Case 3 *(Figs 3-60 to 3-62)*

Clinical situation

The patient is edentulous distal to position 12. Two Regular Platform implants have been placed in positions 13 and 15. Note the offset of screw access holes and the cantilever at position 13 (Figs 3-60 and 3-61).

The biomechanical risk score is 4.0 in this situation. Less than 1 year after prosthesis placement, the prosthetic screws fractured (Fig 3-62, *arrow*).

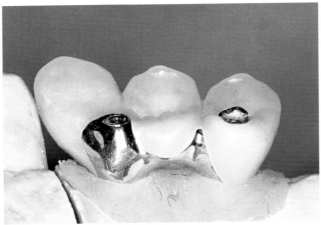

Fig 3-60

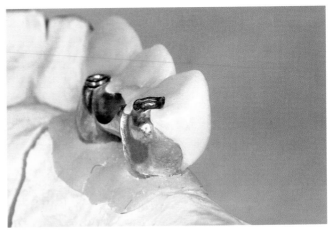

Fig 3-61

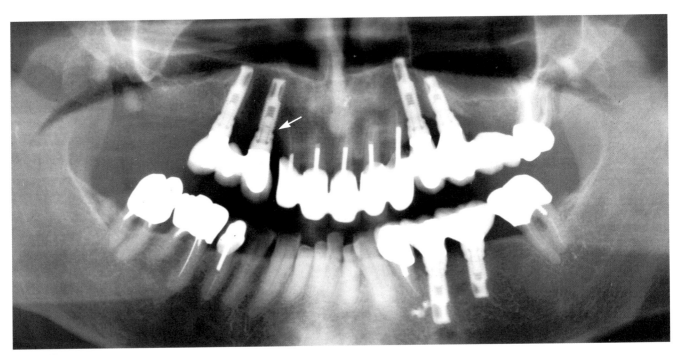

Fig 3-62

Geometric risk factors	Score
Number of implants (N) less than number of root supports (for N<3)	1.0
Use of Wide Platform implants (per implant)	−1.0
Implant connected to a natural tooth	0.5
Implants placed in tripod configuration	−1.0
Presence of a prosthetic extension (per pontic)	1.0
Implants placed offset from the center of the prosthesis	1.0
Excessive height of the restoration	0.5
Occlusal risk factors	**Score**
Bruxism, parafunction, or natural tooth fractures resulting from occlusal factor	2.0
Lateral occlusal contact on the implant-supported prosthesis only	1.0
Lateral occlusal contact essentially on adjacent teeth	−1.0
Bone and implant risk factors	**Score**
Dependence on newly formed bone in the absence of good initial mechanical stability	1.0
Smaller implant diameter than desired	0.5
Technological risk factors	**Score**
Lack of prosthetic fit or nonoptimal screw joint	0.5
Cemented prostheses	0.5

	Okay	Caution	Danger
Biomechanical risk score	<2.0	2.0–3.0	>3.0
Patient's score			4.0

Alarm signals	Score
Repeated loosening of prosthetic or abutment screws	1.0
Repeated fracture of veneering material (resin or ceramic)	1.0
Fracture of prosthetic or abutment screws	2.0
Bone resorption below the first thread of the fixture	1.0

Same patient (Figs 3-63 and 3-64)

A 7-mm Regular Platform implant (4 mm in diameter) was added distally, and the prosthesis was re-made. The biomechanical risk score is reduced to 2.0 and the situation is more favorable. However, the patient should be examined regularly. It is important to ensure that the occlusal scheme does not over-load the implant prosthesis, especially during lateral excursions.

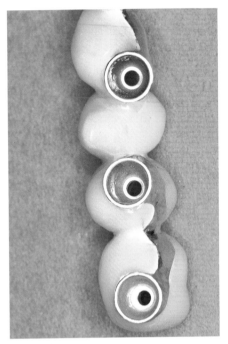

Fig 3-63

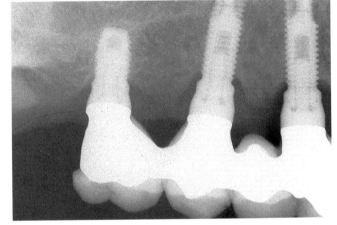

Fig 3-64

Geometric risk factors	Score
Number of implants (N) less than number of root supports (for N<3)	1.0
Use of Wide Platform implants (per implant)	−1.0
Implant connected to a natural tooth	0.5
Implants placed in tripod configuration	−1.0
Presence of a prosthetic extension (per pontic)	1.0
Implants placed offset from the center of the prosthesis	1.0
Excessive height of the restoration	0.5

Occlusal risk factors	Score
Bruxism, parafunction, or natural tooth fractures resulting from occlusal factors	2.0
Lateral occlusal contact on the implant-supported prosthesis only	1.0
Lateral occlusal contact essentially on adjacent teeth	−1.0

Bone and implant risk factors	Score
Dependence on newly formed bone in the absence of good initial mechanical stability	1
Smaller implant diameter than desired	0.5

Technological risk factors	Score
Lack of prosthetic fit or nonoptimal screw joint	0.5
Cemented prostheses	0.5

	Okay	Caution	Danger
Biomechanical risk score	<2.0	2.0–3.0	>3.0
Patient's score		2.0	

Alarm signals	Score
Repeated loosening of prosthetic or abutment screws	1.0
Repeated fracture of veneering material (resin or ceramic)	1.0
Fracture of prosthetic or abutment screws	2.0
Bone resorption below the first thread of the fixture	1.0

Case 4 *(Figs 3-65 to 3-68)*

Clinical situation

A three-unit prosthesis is in positions 34-35-36 in a bruxing patient; two Regular Platform, 3.75-mm diameter implants have been placed in positions 35 and 36 and an extension has been placed at position 34 (Figs 3-65 and 3-66). Several incidences of screw loosening have occurred over the years. Bone resorption appeared around the anterior implant (Fig 3-67) and it was decided to place an extra implant. During the healing period the anterior implant fractured (Fig 3-68, *arrow*).

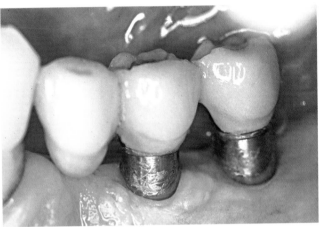

Fig 3-65

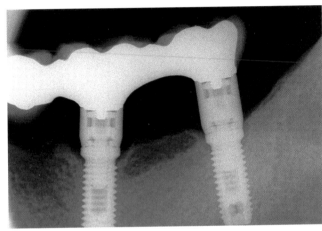

Fig 3-66

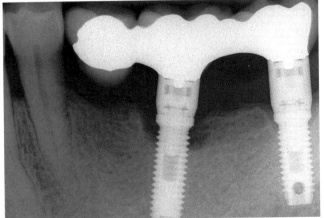

Fig 3-67

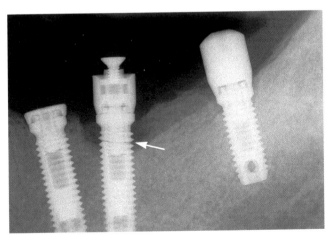

Fig 3-68

Geometric risk factors	Score
Number of implants (N) less than number of root supports (for N<3)	1.0
Use of Wide Platform implants (per implant)	−1.0
Implant connected to a natural tooth	0.5
Implants placed in tripod configuration	−1.0
Presence of a prosthetic extension (per pontic)	1.0
Implants placed offset from the center of the prosthesis	1.0
Excessive height of the restoration	0.5
Occlusal risk factors	**Score**
Bruxism, parafunction, or natural tooth fractures resulting from occlusal factors	2.0
Lateral occlusal contact on the implant-supported prosthesis only	1.0
Lateral occlusal contact essentially on adjacent teeth	−1.0
Bone and implant risk factors	**Score**
Dependence on newly formed bone in the absence of good initial mechanical stability	1.0
Smaller implant diameter than desired	0.5
Technological risk factors	**Score**
Lack of prosthetic fit or nonoptimal screw joint	0.5
Cemented prostheses	0.5

	Okay	Caution	Danger
Biomechanical risk score	<2.0	2.0–3.0	>3.0
Patient's score			4.0

Alarm signals	Score
Repeated loosening of prosthetic or abutment screws	1.0
Repeated fracture of veneering material	1.0
Fracture of prosthetic or abutment screws	2.0
Bone resorption below the first thread of the fixture	1.0

Comment: The patient should have been treated with three implants of 4 mm in diameter. This should have eliminated 2.5 geometric risk factors. Because the patient exhibited bruxism, the placement of the implants in a tripod configuration and/or the use of Wide Platform implants would have been advisable if anatomy allowed. As soon as an alarm occurs in a bruxing patient, corrective actions should be taken.

Suggested readings

Bone tissue

Borsh T, Persovski Z, Binderman I. Mechanical properties of bone-implant interface: An in vitro comparison of the parameters at placement and at 3 months. Int J Oral Maxillofac Implants 1995;10:729-735.

Isidor F. Loss of osseointegration caused by occlusal load of oral implants. A clinical and radiographical study in monkeys. Clin Oral Implants Res 1996;7:143-152.

Quirynen M, Naert I, van Steenberghe D. Fixture design and overload influence marginal bone loss and fixture success in the Brånemark system. Clin Oral Implants Res 1992;3:104-111.

Force distribution

Benzing U, Gall H, Weber H. Biomechanical aspects of two different implant-prosthetic concepts for edentulous maxillae. Int J Oral Maxillofac Implants 1995;10:188-198.

Glantz P-O, Rangert B, Svensson A, Stafford D, Arnvidarson B, Randow K, et al. On clinical loading of osseointegrated implants. Clin Oral Implants Res 1993;4:99-105.

Lundgren D, Laurell L. Biomechanical aspects of fixed bridgework supported by natural teeth and endossous implants. Periodontology 2000 1994;4:23-40.

Mericske-Stern R, Assal P, Buergin W. Simultaneous force measurements in 3 dimensions on oral endosseous implants in vitro and in vivo. Clin Oral Implants Res 1996;7:378-386.

Rangert B, Jemt T, Jörnus L. Forces and moments on Brånemark Implants. Int J Oral Maxillofac Implants 1989;4:241-247.

Richter EJ. In vivo vertical forces on implants. Int J Oral Maxillofac Implants 1995;10:99-108.

Richter EJ, Meier M, Spiekermann H. Implantatsbelastung in vivo. Untersuchungen an implantatgeführten Overdenture-Prosthesen. Z Zahnärztl Implantol 1992;8:36-45.

Occlusal overload

Balshi T. An analysis and management of fractured implants: A clinical report. Int J Oral Maxillofac Implants 1996;11:660-666.

Naert I, Quirynen M, van Steenberghe D, Darius P. A six-year prosthodontic study of 509 consecutively inserted implants for the treatment of partial edentulism. J Prosthet Dent 1992;67:236-245.

Rangert B, Krogh P, Langer B. Bending overload and implant fracture: A resprospective clinical analysis. Int J Oral Maxillofac Implants 1995;10:326-334.

Weinberg L, Kruger B. A comparison of implant/prosthesis loading with four clinical variables. Int J Prosthodont 1995;8:421-433.

Implants connected to natural teeth

Gunne J, Rangert B, Glantz P-O, Svensson A. Functional loads on free-standing and connected implants in 3-unit mandibular bridges opposing complete dentures—an in vivo study. Int J Oral Maxillofac Implants 1997;12:335-341.

Rangert B, Gunne J, Glantz P-O, Svensson A. Vertical load distribution on a 3-unit prosthesis supported by a natural tooth and a single Brånemark implant. An in vivo study. Clin Oral Implants Res 1995;6:40-46.

Rieder C, Parel S. A survey of natural tooth abutment intrusion with implant-connected fixed partial dentures. Int J Periodont Rest Dent 1993;4:335-347.

Sheets C, Earthman JC. Natural tooth intrusion and reversal in implant-assisted prosthesis. J Prosthet Dent 1993;70:513-520.

Screw joints

Jörnéus L, Jemt T, Carlsson L. Loads and design of screw joint for single crowns supported by osseointegrated implants. Int J Oral Maxillofac Implants 1992;7:353-359.

Burguete R, Johns R, King T, Patterson E. Tightening characteristics for screwed joints in osseointegrated dental implants. J Prosthet Dent 1994;71:292-299.

Carr A, Brunski J, Labishak J, Bagley B. Preload comparison between as-received and cast-to implant cylinders. J Dent Res 1993;72(suppl 1):190.

Kallus T, Bessing C. Loose gold screws frequently occur in full-arch fixed prostheses supported by osseointegrated implants after 5 years. Int J Oral Maxillofac Implants 1994;9:169-178.

Guidelines for treatment planning

Brunski J. Biomechanical factors affecting the bone-dental implant interface. Clin Mater 1992;10:153-201.

Bahat O. Treatment planning and placement of implants in the posterior maxillae: Report of 732 consecutive Nobelpharma implants. Int J Oral Maxillofac Implants 1993;8:151-161.

Rangert B. Principe biomécanique du Brånemark System. Implant 1995;1:41-52.

Rangert B, Sullivan R, Jemt T. Load factor control for implants in the posterior partially edentulous segment. Int J Oral Maxillofac Implants 1997;12:360-370.

Treatment of the Edentulous Maxilla

The preliminary examination makes it possible to identify risk patients and implant contraindications. After this analysis is made, the next step is to analyze the specific clinical situation based on the type of edentulism, because each type has its own requirements.

The chapter presents, type by type, proposed implant solutions and their specific limitations and risk factors.

In the tables, the limitations and risk factors are always presented in the same way:

	Okay	Caution	Danger
Risk factor or Limitation	Ideal situation	Situation with moderate risk	Situation with major risk

The presence of several "Cautions" represents a major risk situation and should lead to a reevaluation of the treatment plan.

If the risk factor is found in the "Danger" column, it is advised that the suggested implant solution be rejected.

Note: The definition of occlusal context is given in chapter 1, page 25.

Maxilla: Central Incisor

Clinical situation *(Fig 4-1)*

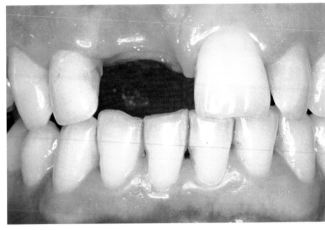

Fig 4-1

Conventional prosthetic solution

- Fixed partial denture
- Resin-bonded prosthesis

Suggested implant solution *(Figs 4-2 to 4-4)*

Regular or Narrow Platform implant with a minimum length of 10 mm and the prosthetic restoration on a CeraOne abutment.

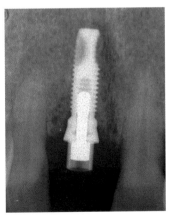

Fig 4-2 The patient is edentulous in position 21. A Regular Platform implant, 3.75 mm in diameter, has been placed. The restoration is made on a CeraOne abutment.

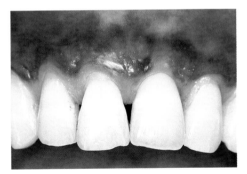

Fig 4-3 Same patient. Final implant restoration 1 year after loading.

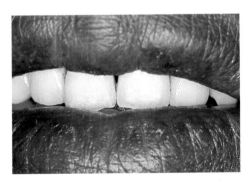

Fig 4-4 Same patient. Appearance when smiling. (Prosthesis by Dr S. Lebars and S. Tissier.)

Note

The implant should be placed in an ideal position in all three dimensions. If the implant axis is palatal to the incisal edge, a screw-retained prosthesis is viable. If the axis is buccal, a cemented-over solution should be considered (Figs 4-5 to 4-8).

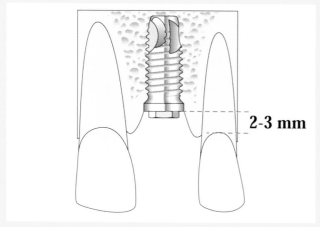

Fig 4-5

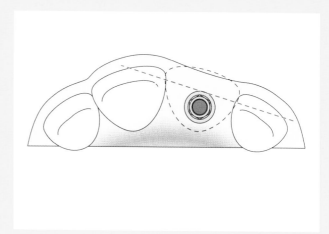

Fig 4-6

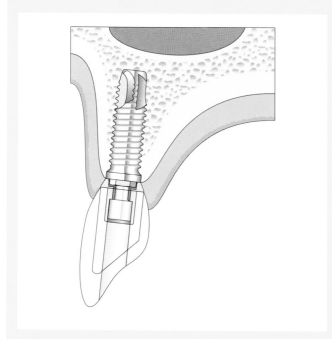

Fig 4-7

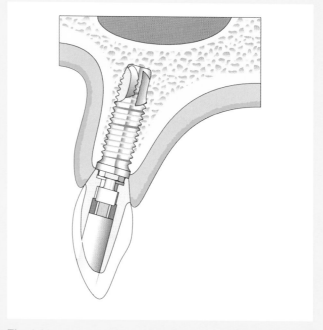

Fig 4-8

Key point

It is essential that a very precise surgical guide be used.

Alternative implant solution *(Figs 4-9 and 4-10)*

If the implant position is not ideal in all three dimensions, or if the peri-implant mucosa is too thin, presenting a risk of abutment visibility, the use of a CerAdapt abutment is recommended.

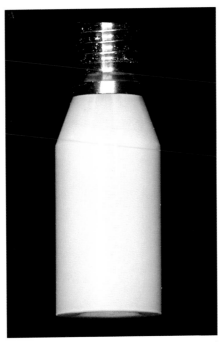

Fig 4-9 CerAdapt abutment fastened to an implant. It should be prepared at the laboratory. The ceramic crown may be fastened directly to the implant, if the implant axis is favorable. If not, a double prosthesis design should be utilized.

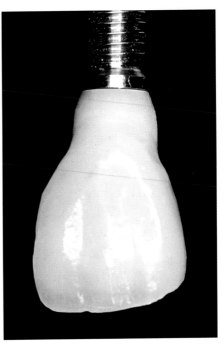

Fig 4-10 Ceramic crown fastened to the CerAdapt abutment. (Prosthesis by N. Milliére.)

Limitations and Risk Factors

Limitation	Okay	Caution	Danger
Mesiodistal distance	>8 mm	7 mm	<6 mm
Thickness of the osseous crest[1]	7 mm	6 mm	<5 mm
Height between the osseous crest and the opposing tooth[2]	7 mm	6 mm	<6 mm

[1] If the osseous crest is too thin, it is possible to enlarge it with bone regeneration or grafting techniques.

[2] The height should be measured from the level of the osseous crest to the occlusal table of the opposing tooth.

Specific Risk Factors	Okay	Caution	Danger
Unrealistic esthetic demands	No		Yes
Smile line[1]	Dental	Gingival	
Vertical bone resorption[2]	No	Considerable	
Gingival morphology	Harmonious		
Mucosal thickness[3]	4–5 mm	<3 mm	
Vestibular concavity	No	Yes	
Nasopalatine canal[4]	Large		
Occlusal context[5]	Favorable	Unfavorable	Unfavorable + offset

[1] The smile line is the first parameter to evaluate before treatment of the edentulous anterior maxilla. If the patient exhibits a large portion of gingiva when smiling, the indication for an implant should be carefully evaluated, especially if any other esthetic risk factor is present.

[2] The presence of substantial vertical bone resorption is a health risk factor for the periodontal and peri-implant tissues. A discrepancy between the marginal bone level of the adjacent teeth and the level of the crest at the implant site represents serious esthetic risk.

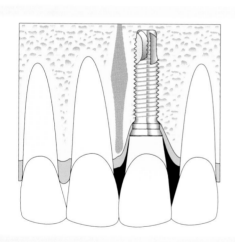

Note

A patient with a gingival smile associated with substantial vertical bone resorption should be considered a patient with a major risk (Fig 4-11).

Fig 4-11

[3] To obtain a satisfactory peri-implant gingival morphology, there should be tissue volume about 20% greater than the estimated need. This surplus allows the prosthodontist to adapt the gingiva to the prosthetic reconstruction.

[4] The diameter of the nasopalatine canal can sometimes be large enough to impede implant placement. The only means of registering the size and position of the canal with sufficient precision is axial computerized tomographic scan sections. It is possible to fill the canal with a bone graft.

[5] A Narrow Platform implant should not be used in the case of parafunction or bruxism.

Note: This checklist is specific for the risk factors involved when the maxillary central incisor is missing. However, before an implant-supported prothesis is planned for in this region, the general checklist should be utilized (see chapter 1, pages 14 and 15).

Note

If the implant is positioned too far labially, there is a risk of mucosal recession and, consequently, an esthetic risk factor is present (Figs 4-12 and 4-13).

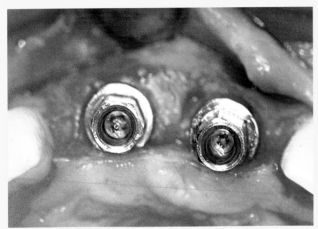

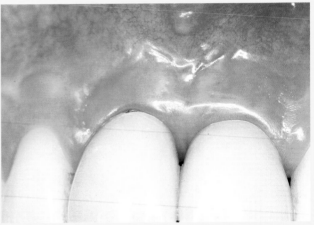

Fig 4-12 Two implants have been placed in positions 11 and 21. CeraOne abutments are in place. Note the slightly too far labial position of the implant in position 11.

Fig 4-13 Same patient at 1-year follow-up. Note the light recession of the mucosa at position 11.

Solutions:
- Place a connective tissue graft.
- Make or remake the prosthesis on a CerAdapt abutment.

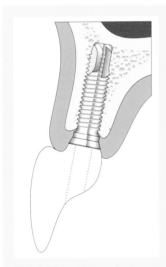

Fig 4-14

Note

If the implant is placed too far palataly, there is a maintenance risk because of the form of the prosthesis. This situation may also lead to screw loosening or debonding of the cemented crown (Fig 4-14).

Note

For esthetic reasons, it is preferable to have the implant placed slightly palatally rather than labially.

Technical note

It is possible to take an impression at the implant level during surgery. This makes it possible to place the definitive abutment and to attach a provisional crown at the second-stage surgery. The adaptation of the mucosa will be more precise.

Maxilla: Lateral Incisor

Clinical situation *(Fig 4-15)*

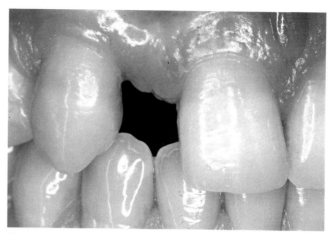

Fig 4-15

Conventional prosthetic solution

- Partial denture
- Resin-bonded prosthesis (Figs 4-16 and 4-17)

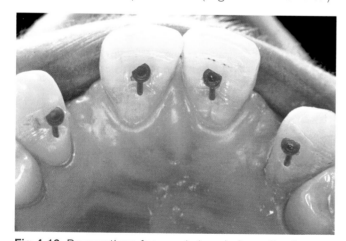

Fig 4-16 Preparations for a resin-bonded prosthesis.

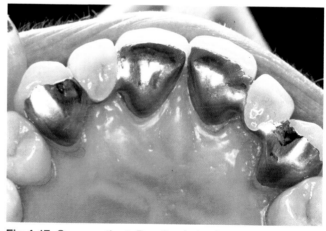

Fig 4-17 Same patient. Prosthesis in place. (Prosthesis by Dr J.-M. Gonzalez, Dr P. Rajzbaum, X. Daniel, and P. Poussin.)

Suggested implant solution

Because the mesiodistal space is limited, placement of a Narrow Platform implant and the prosthetic restoration on a STR abutment should be considered (Figs 4-18 to 4-25).

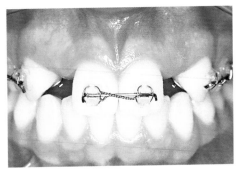

Fig 4-18 Agenesis at positions 12 and 22. Initial situation after completion of orthodontic treatment. (Orthodontic treatment by Dr F. Fontanelle.)

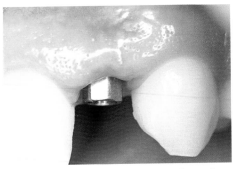

Fig 4-19 Same patient. A CeraOne abutment has been placed on the implant in position 22. Note that the abutment is too wide in this situation.

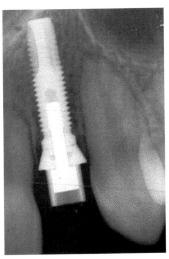

Fig 4-20 Radiographic examination of the CeraOne abutment. Note the proximity to the natural teeth.

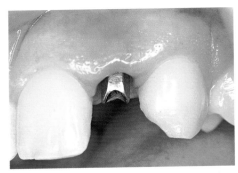

Fig 4-21 Same patient. Clinical view during try-in with a STR abutment. Note that the width is more favorable.

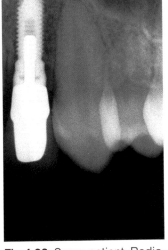

Fig 4-22 Same patient. Radiographic examination of the STR abutment.

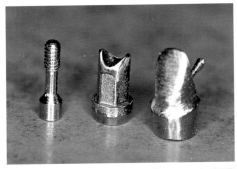

Fig 4-23 Same patient. Prepared STR abutment with screw and metal cap.

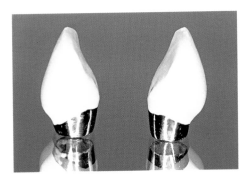

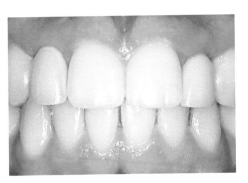

Fig 4-24 Two ceramometal crowns.

Fig 4-25 Same patient. Final situation. (Prosthesis by Dr J. Pillet and P. Amiach.)

Note

Generally, the absence of a maxillary lateral incisor is due to agenesis. The lack of the dental germ suppresses the normal development of the alveolar crest, which leads to a vestibular concavity. In that case, it may be difficult to place the implant along an ideal axis. Bone regeneration or grafting should be considered.

Note

The implant should be placed in an ideal position in all three dimensions. If the implant axis is palatal to the incisal edge, a screw-retained prosthesis is viable. If the axis is buccal, a cemented-over solution should be considered.

Key point

It is essential that a very precise surgical guide be used.

Alternative implant solution

If the implant position is not ideal in all three dimensions, or if the peri-implant mucosa is too thin, presenting a risk of abutment visibility, the TiAdapt or AurAdapt abutment is recommended. It is also possible to use a custom-made abutment (Procera System).

Limitations and risk factors

Limitations	Okay	Caution	Danger
Mesiodistal distance[1]	>7 mm	6 mm	<5 mm
Thickness of the osseous crest[2]	5 mm	4 mm	<4 mm
Height between the osseous crest and the opposing tooth[3]	7 mm	6 mm	<6 mm

[1] The dimensions given are for a Narrow Platform implant. If a Regular Platform implant is used, 1 mm should be added.
[2] If the osseous crest is too thin and/or there is a significant vestibular concavity, bone regeneration or grafting should be considered.
[3] The height should be measured from the level of the osseous crest to the occlusal table of the opposing tooth.

Specific Risk Factors	Okay	Caution	Danger
Unrealistic esthetic demands	No		Yes
Smile line[1]	Dental	Gingival	
Vertical bone resorption[2]	No	Considerable	
Mucosal thickness[3]	4–5 mm	<3 mm	
Vestibular concavity	No	Yes	
Occlusal context	Favorable	Unfavorable	Unfavorable + offset

[1] The smile line is the first parameter to evaluate before treatment of the edentulous anterior maxilla. If the patient exhibits a large portion of gingival smile, the indication for an implant should be carefully evaluated, especially if any other esthetic risk factors are present.

[2] The presence of substantial vertical bone resorption is a health risk factor for the periodontal and peri-implant tissues. A discrepancy between the marginal bone level of the adjacent teeth and the osseous crest at the implant site represents a serious esthetic risk.

[3] To obtain a satisfactory peri-implant gingival morphology, there should be tissue volume about 20% greater than the estimated need. This surplus allows the prosthodontist to adapt the gingiva to the prosthetic reconstruction.

Note: This checklist is specific for the risk factors involved when the maxillary lateral incisor is missing. However, before an implant-supported restoration is planned for in this region, the general checklist should be utilized (see chapter 1, pages 14 and 15).

Technical note

It is possible to take an impression at the implant level during surgery. This makes it possible to place the definitive abutment and to attach a provisional crown at the second stage surgery. The adaptation of the mucosa will in this case be more precise.

Maxilla: Canine

Clinical situation
(Figs 4-26 and 4-27)

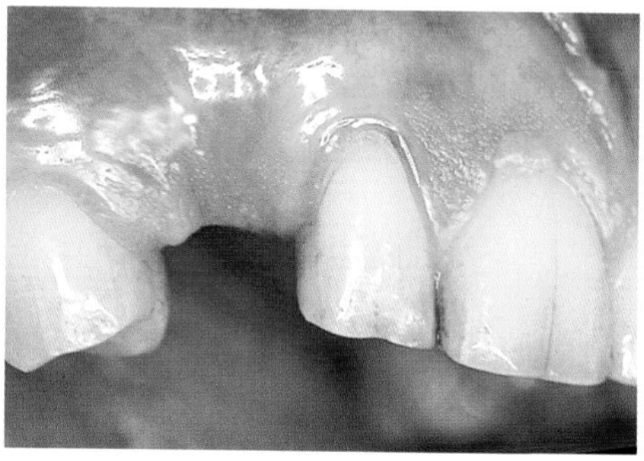

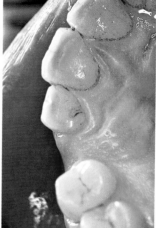

Fig 4-26

Fig 4-27

Conventional prosthetic solution

- Fixed partial denture
- Resin-bonded prosthesis

Suggested implant solution
(Figs 4-28 and 4-29)

Regular Platform implant, 4 mm in diameter, with a minimum length of 10 mm and the prosthetic restoration on a CeraOne abutment.

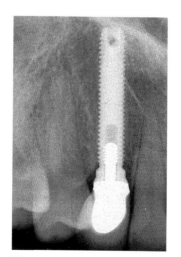

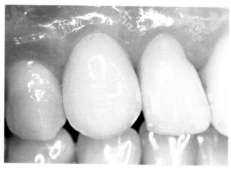

Fig 4-28 Same patient. Radiograph taken 3 years after loading. The restoration is on a CeraOne abutment. (Prosthesis by Dr B. Fleiter and P. Loisel.)

Fig 4-29 Tooth 13 has been replaced with an implant-supported ceramic crown, shown 4 years after loading. Note the esthetic integration of the restoration. (Prosthesis by Dr N. Vincent, X. Daniel, and P. Poussin.)

Note
The implant should be placed in an ideal position in all three dimensions. If the implant axis is palatal to the incisal edge, a screw-retained prosthesis is viable. If the axis is buccal, a cemented-over solution should be considered (see page 69).

Key point
It is essential that a very precise surgical guide be used.

Alternative implant solution

If the implant position is not ideal in all three dimensions or if the peri-implant mucosa is thin, presenting a risk of showing the abutment metal, use of the TiAdapt or the CerAdapt abutment is recommended.

Note: To allow better adaptation of the prosthesis to the gingival contour, the CerAdapt abutment may be indicated to improve the esthetic result.

Limitations and risk factors

Limitation	Okay	Caution	Danger
Mesiodistal distance	>7 mm	6 mm	<6 mm
Thickness of the osseous crest[1]	7 mm	5–6 mm	<4 mm
Height between osseous crest and the opposing tooth[2]	7 mm	6 mm	<6 mm

[1] If the osseous crest is too thin, it is possible to enlarge it with bone regeneration or grafting techniques.
[2] The height should be measured from the level of the osseous crest to the occlusal table of the opposing tooth.

Specific Risk Factors		Okay	Caution	Danger
Unrealistic esthetic demands		No		Yes
Smile line[1]		Dental	Gingival	
Vertical bone resorption[2]		No	Substantial	
Mucosal thickness[3]		4–5 mm	<3 mm	
Implant diameter		≥4 mm	3.75 mm	3.3 mm
Occlusal context[4]	Regular Platform	Favorable	Unfavorable	Unfavorable + canine guidance
	Wide Platform	Unfavorable	Unfavorable + canine guidance	

[1] The smile line is the first parameter to evaluate before treatment of the edentulous anterior maxilla. If the patient exhibits a large portion of gingiva when smiling, the indication for an implant should be carefully evaluated, especially if any other esthetic risk factor is present.

[2] The presence of a substantial vertical bone resorption is a health risk factor for the periodontal and peri-implant tissues. A discrepancy between the marginal bone level of the adjacent teeth and the osseous crest at the implant site represents a serious esthetic risk.

[3] To obtain a satisfactory peri-implant gingival morphology, tissue volume should be about 20% greater than the estimated need. This surplus allows the prosthodontist to adapt the gingiva to the prosthetic reconstruction.

[4] Because implants lack resilience, there is a risk of occlusal overload in the presence of canine guidance, and screw loosening may occur (see Alarm Signals, chapter 3). In a patient who exhibits bruxism or parafunction and canine guidance, use of a Wide Platform implant should be considered, if bone volume and bone density allow.

Note: This checklist is specific for the risk factors involved when the maxillary canine is missing. However, before an implant-supported restoration is planned for in this region, the general checklist should be utilized (see chapter 1, pages 14 and 15).

Technical note

It is possible to take an impression at the implant level during surgery. This makes it possible to place the definitive abutment and to attach a provisional crown at the second-stage surgery. The adaptation of the mucosa will be more precise.

Maxilla: Premolar

Clinical situation *(Fig 4-30)*

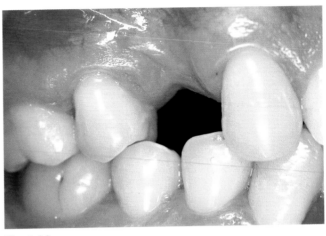

Fig 4-30

Conventional prosthetic solution

- Partial denture
- Resin-bonded prosthesis (Fig 4-31)

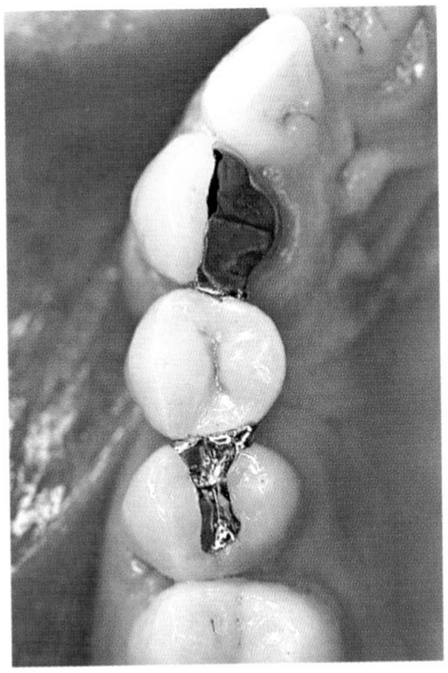

Suggested implant solution *(Figs 4-32 to 4-34)*

Regular Platform implant, 4 mm in diameter, with a minimum length of 10 mm and the prosthetic restoration on a CeraOne abutment.

Fig 4-31 Occlusal view of a resin-bonded prosthesis.

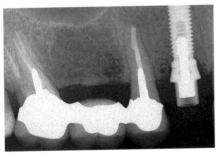

Fig 4-32 Tooth 14 has been replaced with an implant, shown during the placement of the CeraOne abutment.

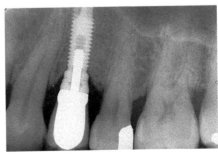

Fig 4-33 Tooth 24 has been replaced with an implant prosthesis, shown 1 year after loading.

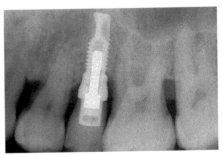

Fig 4-34 Tooth 25 has been replaced with an implant prosthesis, shown 3 years after loading. The patient had severe periodontal disease, which was treated before implant placement. Note the stability of the peri-implant bone level. (Periodontal treatment by Dr J.-L. Giovannoli.)

Alternative implant solution

If the width of the osseous crest allows and the bone density is favorable, the use of a wide implant is recommended. For prosthetic reasons, sometimes the Regular Platform 5-mm-diameter implant should be considered. If the peri-implant mucosa is thin, presenting a risk of showing the abutment metal, the use of CerAdapt is recommended.

Limitations and risk factors

Limitation	Okay	Caution	Danger
Mesiodistal distance[1]	>7 mm	6 mm	<6 mm
Thickness of the osseous crest[2]	7 mm	6 mm	<5 mm
Height between the osseous crest and the opposing tooth[3]	7 mm	6 mm	<6 mm

[1] Dimensions are given for a Regular Platform implant. If a wide platform or 5-mm implant is used, 1 mm should be added.
[2] If the osseous crest is too thin, it is possible to enlarge it with bone regeneration or grafting techniques.
[3] The height should be measured from the level of the osseous crest to the occlusal table of the opposing tooth.

Specific Risk Factors		Okay	Caution	Danger
Position of sinus			Anterior	
Bone density[1]		Type I-II-III	Type IV	
Vestibular concavity		No	Yes	
Implant diameter		≥4 mm	3.75 mm	3.3 mm
Occlusal context[2]	Regular Platform	Favorable	Unfavorable	Unfavorable + lateral contacts
	Wide Platform	Unfavorable	Unfavorable + lateral contacts	

[1] Under the sinus, the bone often has a low density. The use of larger-diameter implants should, therefore, be considered. The healing time should be prolonged in situations with Type IV bone.
[2] Because implants are considerably more rigid than teeth, there is a risk that the implants may absorb a larger share of the load when mixed with natural teeth. Therefore, lateral occlusal contacts on the implant crown should be avoided and the cuspal inclination should be low.

Note: This checklist is specific for the risk factors involved when the maxillary premolar is missing. However, before an implant-supported restoration is planned for in this region, the general checklist should be utilized (see chapter 1, pages 14 and 15).

Technical note

It is possible to take an impression at the implant level during surgery. This makes it possible to place the definitive abutment and to attach a provisional crown at the second-stage surgery. The adaptation of the mucosa will be more precise.

Maxilla: Molar

Clinical situation *(Fig 4-35)*

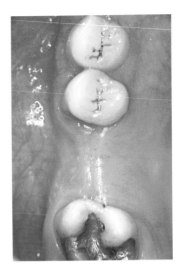

Fig 4-35

Conventional prosthetic solution

■ Fixed partial denture
■ Resin-bonded prosthesis (Figs 4-36 and
4-37)

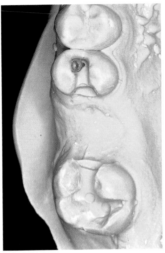

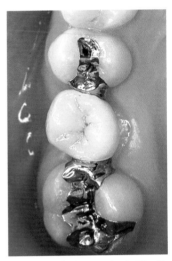

Fig 4-36 Laboratory cast. The patient is edentulous in position 16.

Fig 4-37 Same patient. Tooth 16 is replaced with a resin-bonded prosthesis. (Prosthesis by Dr J.-M. Gonzalez, Dr P. Rajzbaum, X. Daniel, and P. Poussin.)

Suggested implant solution *(Fig 4-38)*

Wide Platform implant with a minimum length of 10 mm and the prosthetic restoration on a CeraOne abutment.

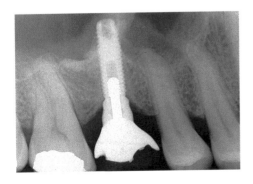

Fig 4-38 Same patient. Radiograph taken at 7 years follow-up after placement of the acrylic resin metal crown. Bone grafting was performed before implant placement. Today, a Wide Platform implant would be used.

Note
The implant axis should be directed through the center of the occlusal table to increase the biomechanical resistance of the restoration.

Alternative implant solution

If the mesiodistal space is too large (>12 mm), it is possible to use two Regular Platform implants to increase the biomechanical resistance of the restoration.

Limitations and risk factors

Limitation	Okay	Caution	Danger
Mesiodistal distance[1]	>8 mm	7 mm	<7 mm
Thickness of the osseous crest[2]	8 mm	6 mm	<5 mm
Height between the osseous crest and the opposing tooth[3]	7 mm	6 mm	<6 mm

[1] Dimensions are given for a Wide Platform implant. If a Regular Implant is used, 1 mm should be subtracted.
[2] If the osseous crest is too thin, it is possible to enlarge it with bone regeneration or grafting techniques.
[3] The height should be measured from the level of osseous crest to the occlusal table of the opposing tooth.

Specific Risk Factors	Okay	Caution	Danger
Position of sinus		Low	
Bone density[1]	Type I-II-III	Type IV	
Mesiodistal space[2]	10 mm	>12 mm	
Implant length	10 mm	8.5 mm	<7 mm
Implant diameter	5 mm	4 mm	3.75 mm
Occlusal context[3]	Favorable	Unfavorable	Unfavorable + lateral contact

[1] Under the sinus, the bone often has a low density. The use of larger-diameter implants should, therefore, be considered. The healing time should be prolonged in situations with Type IV bone.
[2] If the mesiodistal space is 12 mm or more, it is possible to place two Regular Platform implants.
[3] Because implants are considerably more rigid than teeth, there is a risk that the implants may absorb a larger share of the load when mixed with natural teeth. Therefore, lateral occlusal contacts on the implant crown should be avoided and the cuspal inclination should be low.

Note: This checklist is specific for the risk factors involved when the maxillary molar is missing. However, before an implant-supported restoration is planned for in this region, the general checklist should be utilized (see chapter 1, pages 14 and 15).

Maxilla: Anterior, Two Teeth Missing

Clinical situation
(Figs 4-39 and 4-40)

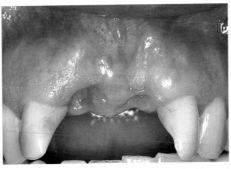

Fig 4-39 The patient has lost teeth 11 and 12 in an accident. Despite the bone defect, the situation is favorable because the patient has a favorable smile line and the available mesiodistal space is sufficient (the restoration is presented in Fig 4-41 and following).

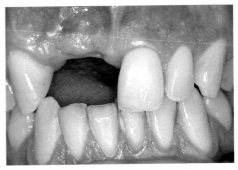

Fig 4-40 The patient has lost teeth 11 and 12 in an accident. Because of the small available mesiodistal space, the situation is complex. The regeneration of the papilla between teeth 11 and 12 is not likely to occur.

Conventional prosthetic solution

▢ Fixed partial denture
▢ Removable partial denture

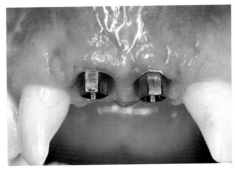

Fig 4-41 The patient has lost teeth 11 and 12 to trauma. Two 13-mm Regular Platform implants have been inserted. Clinical situation after placement of the CeraOne abutment.

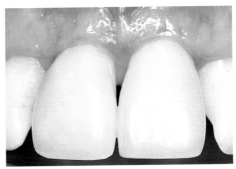

Fig 4-42 Same patient with the provisional crowns in the mouth.

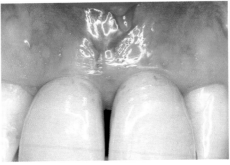

Fig 4-43 Same patient 1 year after placement of the final ceramometal crowns. (Prosthesis by Dr P.-E. Crubillé and C. Laval.)

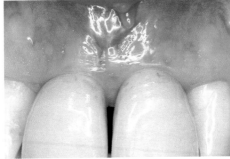

Fig 4-44 Same patient. Radiographic examination 18 months after loading. (The surgical phase is presented in Figs 6-34 to 6-36 on page 162.)

Suggested implant solution

Edentulous positions 11 and 21 (Figs 4-41 to 4-44): Two Regular Platform implants on single-crown restorations (CeraOne, CerAdapt, or TiAdapt).

Edentulous positions 11 and 12 or 21 and 22 (Fig 4-45): One Regular and one Narrow Platform implant or two Narrow Platform implants with single-crown restorations (CeraOne, CerAdapt, TiAdapt, or STR).

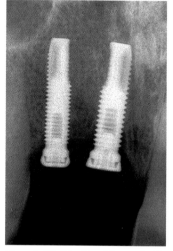

Fig 4-45 Teeth 21 and 22 have been replaced with implants. Note the use of a Narrow Platform implant (3.3 mm in diameter) for replacement of the lateral incisor.

> **Note**
>
> A good esthetic result depends on the possibility of obtaining papillary regeneration between the two implants (see chapter 2).

> **Note**
>
> The replacement of a central incisor and a lateral incisor with implant-supported prostheses represents a major esthetic challenge and should be approached with great care.

> **Key point**
>
> It is essential that a very precise surgical guide be used.

Limitations and risk factors

Limitation	Okay	Caution	Danger
Mesiodistal distance	15 mm	<15 mm	<13 mm
Thickness of the osseous crest[1]	7 mm	6 mm	<6 mm
Height between the osseous crest and the opposing tooth[2]	7 mm	5 mm	<5 mm

[1] If the osseous crest is too thin, it is possible to enlarge it with bone regeneration or grafting techniques.
[2] The height should be measured from the level of osseous crest to the occlusal table of the opposing tooth. If a CeraOne abutment is used, the height must be a minimum of 7 mm.

Specific Risk Factors	Okay	Caution	Danger
Unrealistic esthetic demands	No	Yes	
Smile line[1]	Dental	Gingival	
Vertical bone resorption[2]	No	Substantial	
Gingival morphology	Harmonious		
Mucosal thickness[3]	4–5 mm	<3 mm	
Vestibular concavity	No	Yes	
Nasopalatine canal[4]		Large	
Occlusal context	Favorable	Unfavorable	Unfavorable + offset/cantilever

[1] The smile line is the first parameter to evaluate before treatment of the edentulous anterior maxilla. If the patient exhibits a large portion of gingiva when smiling, the indication for an implant should be carefully considered, especially if any other esthetic risk factor is present.

[2] The presence of substantial vertical bone resorption is a health risk factor for the periodontal and peri-implant tissues. A discrepancy between the marginal bone level of the adjacent teeth and the level of the crest at the implant site represents a serious esthetic risk.

[3] To obtain satisfactory peri-implant gingival morphology, tissue volume should be about 20% greater than the estimated need. This surplus allows the prosthodontist to adapt the gingiva to the prosthetic reconstruction.

[4] The diameter of the nasopalatine canal can sometimes be large enough to impede implant placement. The only means of registering the size and position of the canal with sufficient precision is axial computerized tomographic sections. It is possible to fill the canal with a bone graft. The use of Narrow Platform implants should be considered.

Note: This checklist is specific for the risk factors involved when two teeth are missing from the anterior maxilla. However, before an implant-supported restoration is planned for in this region, the general checklist should be utilized (see chapter 1, pages 14 and 15).

Technical note

It is possible to take an impression at the implant level during surgery. This makes it possible to place the definitive abutments and to attach provisional crowns at the second-stage surgery. The adaptation of the mucosa will be more precise.

Maxilla: Anterior, Three Teeth Missing

Clinical situation *(Figs 4-46 and 4-47)*

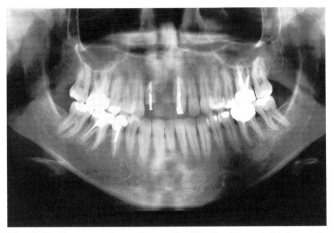

Fig 4-46 Panoramic radiograph. Teeth 12 and 21 have to be extracted. An implant solution is foreseen. (Radiography by Drs G. Pasquet and R. Cavezian.)

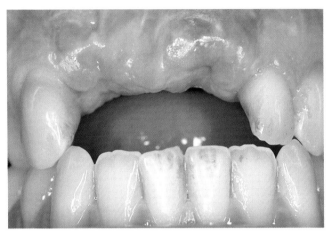

Fig 4-47 Same patient after extraction of teeth 12 and 21.

Conventional prosthetic solution

- Fixed partial denture
- Removable partial denture

Suggested implant solution

This situation can be treated with one fixed partial denture or with three single crowns.

● Two Regular Platform implants with a prosthetic bridge reconstruction on EsthetiCone or MirusCone abutments (Figs 4-48 and 4-49).

● Three Regular or Narrow Platform implants with three single crowns on CeraOne, CerAdapt, or TiAdapt abutments.

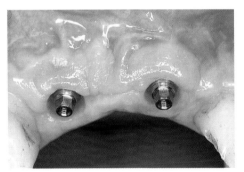

Fig 4-48 Same patient. Two implants have been placed in positions 12 and 21. Appearance at placement of the EsthetiCone abutments.

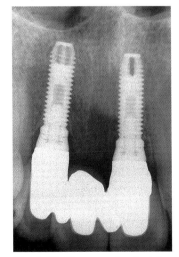

Fig 4-49 Same patient at the 3-year follow-up.

Note

To prevent the implants from being too close, it is preferable that a Narrow Platform implant be used to replace the lateral incisors.

Alternative implant solution

Two Regular Platform implants with a prosthetic bridge on two MirusCone abutments and an extension (Figs 4-50 to 4-54).

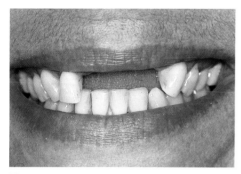

Fig 4-50 Initial situation. The patient has lost teeth 11, 21, and 22 to trauma. Visualization of the smile line.

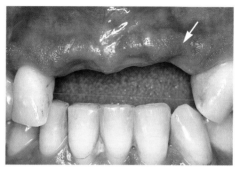

Fig 4-51 Same patient. Extensive bone loss impedes placement of an implant in position 22. Note the horizontal bone loss *(arrow)*. The area is not visible when the patient is smiling, and it was decided not to place a bone graft before the restoration.

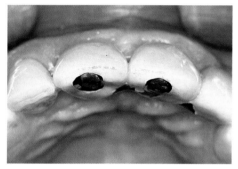

Fig 4-52 Same patient. Occlusal view of the final prosthesis. Note the extension in position 22.

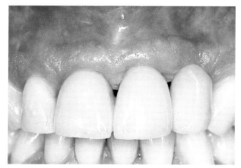

Fig 4-53 Same patient. Final prosthesis 1 year after placement. (Prosthesis by Dr C. Finelle, X. Daniel, and P. Poussin.)

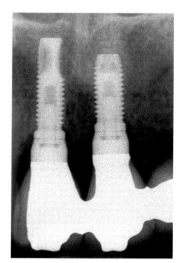

Fig 4-54 Same patient 1 year after loading.

Note

It is important to avoid occlusal contact on the extension during excursive movements of the mandible. Use of a 4-mm-diameter implant as distal support should be considered (Figs 4-55 to 4-57).

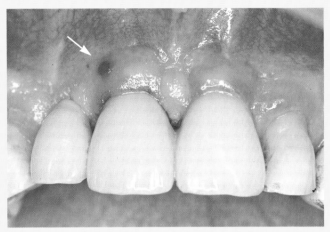

Fig 4-55 Two-year follow-up after loading. The patient consults for pain at the implant site in position 11. Note the fistula located distal to position 11 *(arrow)*.

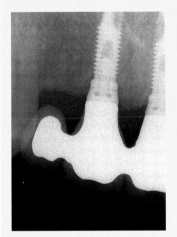

Fig 4-56 Same patient. Retroalveolar radiograph. No bone loss is visible. The prosthesis and the abutment seem to be in place. The prosthesis was removed and the abutment screw and prosthesis were examined. The abutment screw of implant in position 11 was loose. The abutment was disinfected, and the abutment screw was changed.

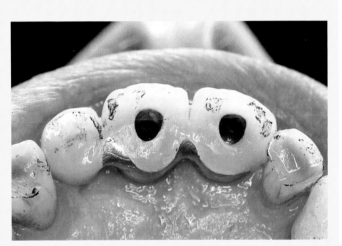

Fig 4-57 Same patient. Occlusal examination. Note the contact at the extension. Note the abrasion on the adjacent teeth, which provides evidence of an unfavorable occlusal context. If the occlusal contact on the extension not suppressed during excursive jaw motion, the complication is likely to be reproduced.

Limitations and risk factors

Limitation	Okay	Caution	Danger
Mesiodistal distance	21 mm	19 mm	<18 mm
Thickness of the osseous crest[1]	7 mm	6 mm	<5 mm
Height between the osseous crest and the opposing tooth[2]	7 mm	6 mm	<5 mm

[1] If the osseous crest is too thin, it is possible to enlarge it with bone regeneration or grafting techniques.

[2] The height should be measured from the level of the osseous crest to the occlusal table of the opposing tooth. If a CeraOne abutment is used, the height must be a minimum of 7 mm.

Specific Risk Factors	Okay	Caution	Danger
Unrealistic esthetic demands	No	Yes	
Smile line[1]	Dental	Gingival	
Vertical bone resorption[2]	No	Substantial	
Gingival morphology	Harmonious		
Mucosal thickness[3]	4–5 mm	<3 mm	
Vestibular concavity	No	Yes	
Nasopalatine canal[4]		Large	
Occlusal context	Favorable	Unfavorable	Unfavorable + offset/cantilever

[1] The smile line is the first parameter to evaluate before treatment of the edentulous anterior maxilla. If the patient exhibits a large portion of gingiva when smiling, the indication for an implant should be carefully evaluated, especially if any other esthetic risk factors are present.

[2] The presence of substantial vertical bone resorption is a health risk factor for the periodontal and peri-implant tissues. A discrepancy between the marginal bone level of the adjacent teeth and the level of the crest at the implant site represents a serious esthetic risk.

[3] To obtain a satisfactory peri-implant gingival morphology, tissue volume should be 20% greater than the estimated need. This surplus allows the prosthodontist to adapt the gingiva to the prosthetic reconstruction.

[4] The diameter of the nasopalatine canal can sometimes be large enough to impede implant placement. The only means of registering the size and position of the canal with sufficient precision is axial computerized tomographic sections. It is possible to fill the canal with a bone graft. Use of a Narrow Platform implant should be considered.

Note: This checklist is specific for the risk factors involved when three teeth are missing in the anterior maxilla. However, before an implant-supported restoration is planned for in this region, the general checklist should be utilized (see chapter 1, pages 14 and 15).

Technical note

It is possible to take an impression at the implant level during surgery. This makes it possible to place definitive abutments and to attach provisional crowns at the second-stage surgery. The adaptation of the mucosa will be more precise.

Maxilla: Anterior, Four Teeth Missing

Clinical situation (Figs 4-58 and 4-59)

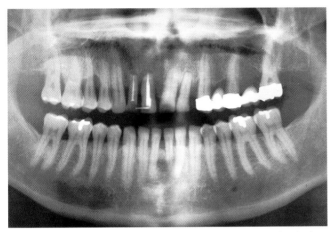

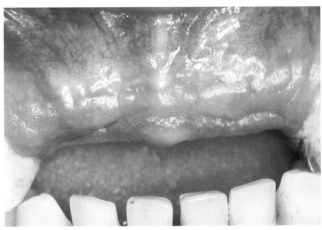

Fig 4-58 Panoramic radiograph. The patient is being treated for periodontal disease. The four maxillary incisors should be extracted. (Radiograph by Drs G. Pasquet and R. Cavezian.)

Fig 4-59 Same patient 2 months postextraction.

Conventional prosthetic solution

- Fixed partial denture
- Removable partial denture (Fig 4-60)

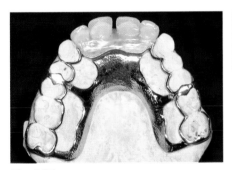

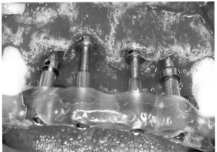

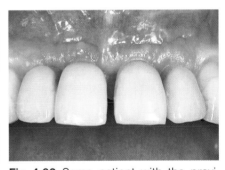

Fig 4-60

Fig 4-61 Same patient as in Fig 4-58. Clinical view during implant placement. Note the use of a very precise surgical guide (see chapter 6). To place the implants at the same depth, a bone regeneration technique is used.

Fig 4-62 Same patient with the provisional restoration 6 months after loading. (Prosthesis by Dr J.-M. Gonzalez, Dr P. Rajzbaum, X. Daniel, and P. Poisson.)

Suggested implant solution

- Four Regular or Narrow Platform implants with single crowns on CeraOne, CerAdapt, or TiAdapt abutments (Figs 4-61 and 4-62).

● Three Regular Platform implants with a prosthetic bridge reconstruction on MirusCone, EsthetiCone, or TiAdapt abutments.

To prevent the implants from being too close, it is preferable that a Narrow Platform implant be used to replace the lateral incisors.

Alternative implant solution

● Two Regular Platform 4-mm-diameter implants and a prosthetic bridge reconstruction with two extensions on MirusCone abutments (Figs 4-63 to 4-66).

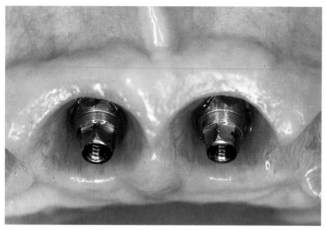

Fig 4-63 Teeth 12, 11, 21, and 22 have been lost to periodontal disease. Two implants have been placed in positions 11 and 21. Use of two EsthetiCone abutments.

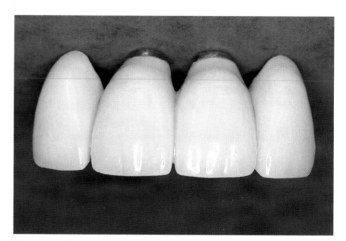

Fig 4-64 Same patient. Ceramometal bridge.

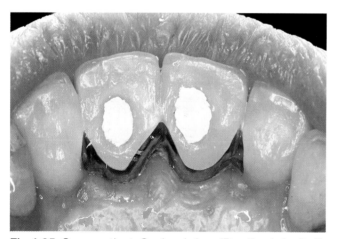

Fig 4-65 Same patient. Occlusal view. (Prosthesis by Dr C. Knaffo-Bellity and J. Dhont.)

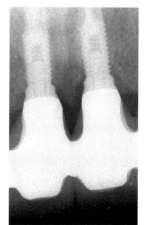

Fig 4-66 Radiograph taken 3 years after loading. The situation is stable. This circumstance, however, should be considered to be associated with a certain risk. The bone loss around implant 21 was detected at the abutment connection.

Note

It is important to avoid occlusal contact on the extension during excursive movements of the mandible. Use of 4-mm-diameter implants should be considered. This situation entails a certain risk.

● Two Regular Platform implants (if possible, 4 mm in diameter) and a prosthetic bridge reconstruction on MirusCone or TiAdapt abutments.

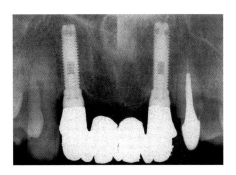

Fig 4-67 The patient is edentulous in positions 12 to 22. Two implants have been placed. A prosthesis was made. Radiograph taken 2 years after loading.

Limitations and risk factors

Limitation	Okay	Caution	Danger
Mesiodistal distance	28 mm	25 mm	<24 mm
Thickness of the osseous crest[1]	7 mm	6 mm	<5 mm
Height between the osseous crest and the opposing tooth[2]	7 mm	6 mm	<5 mm

[1] If the osseous crest is too thin, it is possible to enlarge it with bone regeneration or grafting techniques.
[2] The height should be measured from the level of osseous crest to the occlusal table of the opposing tooth. If a CeraOne abutment is used, the height must be a minimum of 7 mm.

Specific Risk Factors	Okay	Caution	Danger
Unrealistic esthetic demands	No	Yes	
Smile line[1]	Dental	Gingival	
Vertical bone resorption[2]		No	Substantial
Gingival morphology	Harmonious		
Mucosal thickness[3]	4–5 mm	<3 mm	
Palatal nasal canal[4]		Large	
Vestibular concavity	No	Yes	
Number and positions of implants (see table on next page)			

[1] The smile line is the first parameter to evaluate before treatment of the edentulous anterior maxilla. If the patient exhibits a large portion of gingiva when smiling, the indication for an implant should be carefully evaluated, especially if any other esthetic risk factors are present.
[2] The presence of substantial vertical bone resorption is a health risk factor for the periodontal and peri-implant tissues. A discrepancy between the marginal bone level of the adjacent teeth and the level of the crest at the implant site represents a serious esthetic risk.
[3] To obtain satisfactory peri-implant gingival morphology, tissue volume should be about 20% greater than the estimated need. This surplus allows the prosthodontist to adapt the gingiva to the prosthetic reconstruction.
[4] The diameter of the palatal nasal canal can sometimes be large enough to impede implant placement. The only means of registering the size and position of the canal with sufficient precision is axial computerized tomographic sections. It is possible to fill the canal with a bone graft. Use of a Narrow Platform Implant should be considered.

Occlusal risk factors	Okay	Caution	Danger
NP RP RP NP	Favorable occlusal context	Unfavorable occlusal context	Unfavorable occlusal context + offset
NP RP RP RP	All situations		
RP RP	Favorable occlusal context	Unfavorable occlusal context	Unfavorable occlusal context + offset
RP RP	No contacts at extensions	Contacts at extensions	Unfavorable occlusal context

Note: This checklist is specific for the risk factors involved when four teeth are missing in the anterior maxilla. However, before an implant-supported restoration is planned for in this region, the general checklist should be utilized (see chapter 1, pages 14 and 15).

Technical note

It is possible to take an impression at the implant level during surgery. This makes it possible to place definitive abutments and to attach provisional crowns at the second-stage surgery. The adaptation of the mucosa will be more precise.

Maxilla: Posterior, Two Teeth Missing

Clinical situation *(Figs 4-68 and 4-69)*

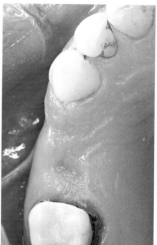

Conventional prosthetic solution

- Fixed partial denture
- Removable partial denture

Fig 4-68   **Fig 4-69**

Suggested implant solution

Edentation	Implants
2 premolars (2 root supports)	2 Regular Platform, 4 mm in diameter
1 premolar + 1 molar (3 root supports)	3 Regular Platform or 1 Regular + 1 Wide Platform
2 molars (4 root supports)	3 Regular Platform or 2 Wide Platform

It is suggested that two teeth missing between natural teeth be replaced by single-tooth abutments, CeraOne, or TiAdapt (Fig 4-70), and that two splinted teeth on MirusCone or TiAdapt abutments be used for the free-end situation (Fig 4-71). Splinting is recommended in all situations in which the position or inclination of the implant axis is unfavorable.

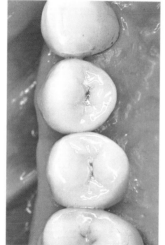
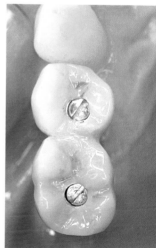

Fig 4-70 *(left)* Occlusal view. The space in positions 14 and 15 has been filled with two single crowns on CerAdapt abutments. (Prosthesis by Dr J.-M. Gonzalez, Dr P. Rajzbaum, X. Daniel, and P. Poussin.)

Fig 4-71 *(right)* Occlusal view. The free-end situation in positions 14 and 15 has been restored with two splinted crowns. The presence of a large sinus prevents placement of a third implant. Note that a molar has been placed in position 15 to increase the occlusal contact surface. (Prosthesis by Dr J.-M. Gonzalez, Dr P. Rajzbaum, and C. Laval.)

Alternative implant solution

Sometimes, because of a prominent sinus, it is not possible to place the minimum of two implants in a free-end situation. When only a single implant can be placed posteriorly to the distal tooth, a prosthetic bridge may be made to connect the implant to that tooth. Such connection should be rigid to ensure distribution of the occlusal forces between the implant and the tooth.

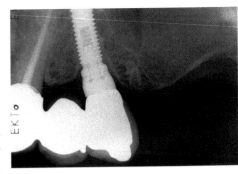

Fig 4-72 Radiograph taken 4 years after loading. Because of the position of the sinus, only one implant was placed. The connection to the canine is rigid. Note the stable bone level around the implant. However, this situation should be considered to be associated with a risk.

Note

This situation should be considered to entail a certain biomechanical risk (see the biomechanical checklist in chapter 3). Wide Platform implants should be considered in this situation because of their greater load capacity.

Limitations and risk factors

Limitation	Okay	Caution	Danger
Mesiodistal distance[1]	15 mm	>14 mm	
Thickness of the osseous crest[2]	7 mm	6 mm	<5 mm
Height between the osseous crest and the opposing tooth[3]	7 mm	6 mm	<5 mm

[1] The dimensions given are for Regular Platform implants. If Wide Platform implants are used, 2 mm should be added.
[2] If the osseous crest is too thin, it is possible to enlarge it with bone regeneration or grafting techniques. In this situation, the healing time should be prolonged.
[3] The height should be measured from the level of osseous crest to the occlusal table of the opposing tooth. If a CeraOne abutment is used, the height must be a minimum of 7 mm.

Specific Risk Factors	Okay	Caution	Danger
Position of sinus		Anterior and low	
Bone density[1]	Type I-II-III	Type IV	
Occlusal context[2]	Favorable	Unfavorable	Unfavorable + offset/extension
Implant diameter	≥4 mm	3.75 mm	3.3 mm

[1] Under the sinus, the bone often has a low density. The use of larger-diameter implants should, therefore, be considered. The healing time should be prolonged in situations with Type IV bone.
[2] Because implants are considerably more rigid than teeth, lateral occlusal contacts on the implant crown should be avoided and the cuspal inclination should be low in the posterior region.

Note: This checklist is specific for the risk factors involved when two teeth are missing in the posterior maxilla. However, before an implant-supported restoration is planned for in this region, the general checklist should be utilized (see chapter 1, pages 14 and 15).

Maxilla: Posterior, Three or Four Teeth Missing

Clinical situation *(Fig 4-73)*

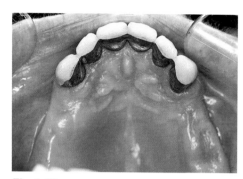

Conventional prosthetic solution *(Figs 4-74 and 4-75)*

■ Removable partial denture

Fig 4-73

Fig 4-74 (Prosthesis by Dr J.-M. Gonzalez, Dr P. Rajzbaum, C. Laval, and C. Millet.)

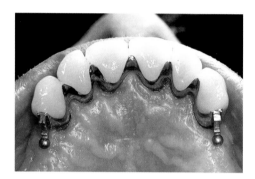

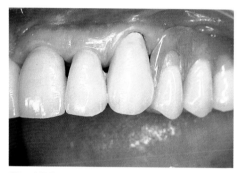

Fig 4-75

Suggested implant solution *(Figs 4-76 and 4-77)*

Minimum of three Regular Platform implants with a fixed partial denture (three to four crowns) on MirusCone abutments. Use of Regular Platform implants, 4 mm in diameter, or Wide Platform implants should be considered.

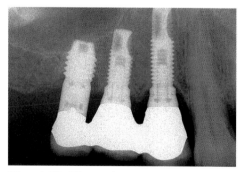

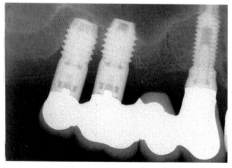

Fig 4-76 Three implants have been placed to replace the teeth lost distal to position 13. Shown is the situation 3 years after loading. Note the use of Regular Platform implants 5 mm in diameter and 6 mm long posteriorly. Note the stability of the peri-implant bone. Note the reduction of the occlusal surface in position 16. (Prosthesis by Dr D. Vilbert and S. Tissier.)

Fig 4-77 Three implants have been placed to replace the teeth lost distal to position 13. Shown is the situation 4 years after loading. Note the use of two Regular Platform implants 5 mm in diameter and 6 mm long posteriorly. Note the stability of the peri-implant bone. (Prosthesis by Dr D. Vilbert and Mr S. Tissier.)

Alternative implant solution

Sometimes only two implants can be placed. This situation is far from ideal and should be considered to entail a moderate to substantial biomechanical risk. Use of Wide Platform implants should be considered in this situation because of their greater load capacity.

> **Note**
> Connection of two implants with one or more natural teeth is not recommended. The splint can be considered an unsupported extension to the implant prosthesis, because the implants have a much stiffer anchorage than the teeth. This situation represents a substantial biomechanical risk.

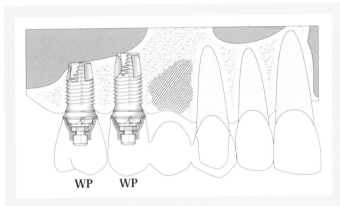

WP   WP

Note
If only two implants can be placed, it is preferable to connect only one to the teeth and to place a single crown on the other. The bending flexibility of the implant will compensate for the mobility of the tooth. Use of Wide Platform implants is recommended in this situation (Fig 4-78).

Fig 4-78

Limitations and risk factors

Limitation	Okay	Caution	Danger
Thickness of the osseous crest[1,2]	7 mm	6 mm	<5 mm
Height between the osseous crest and the opposing tooth[3]	7 mm	6 mm	<6 mm

[1] The dimensions given are for Regular Platform. If Wide Platform or 5-mm-diameter implants are used, 1 mm should be added.
[2] If the osseous crest is too thin, it is possible to enlarge it with bone regeneration or grafting techniques. In this situation, the healing time should be prolonged.
[3] The height should be measured from the level of osseous crest to the occlusal table of the opposing tooth. If a CeraOne abutment is used, the height must be a minimum of 7 mm.

Specific Risk Factors	Okay	Caution	Danger
Bone density[1]	Type I-II-III	Type IV	
Position of sinus[2]		Anterior and low	
Number/positions of implants, occlusion (see table on next page)			

[1] Under the sinus, the bone often hase a low density. The use of larger- diameter implants should, therefore, be considered. The healing time should be prolonged in situations with Type IV bone.
[2] When the sinus volume does not allow placement of an implant under favorable conditions, a sinus-grafting procedure may be considered.

Occlusal risk factors for three teeth		Okay	Caution	Danger
 RP RP RP		Moderately unfavorable occlusal context	Highly unfavorable occlusal context	
 WP WP WP		Highly unfavorable occlusal context		
 RP RP		Favorable occlusal context	Moderately unfavorable occlusal context	Highly unfavorable occlusal context
 WP WP		Moderately unfavorable occlusal context	Highly unfavorable occlusal context	
 WP WP WP		Favorable occlusal context	Moderately unfavorable occlusal context	Highly unfavorable occlusal context

Occlusal risk factors for three teeth		Okay	Caution	Danger
		Moderately unfavorable occlusal context	Highly unfavorable occlusal context	
WP WP				
			Favorable occlusal context	Moderately unfavorable occlusal context
RP RP				
		Favorable occlusal context	Moderately unfavorable occlusal context	Highly unfavorable occlusal context
WP WP				

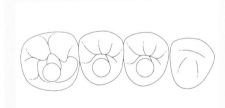

Note

If the implants are placed offset from the center of the occlusal table, at the position of the buccal or lingual cusps, the recommendation is moved one step to the right (less favorable).

Okay	⟶	Caution
Caution	⟶	Danger

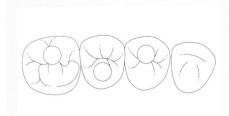

Note

If the implants are placed in a tripod configuration, the recommendation is moved one step to the left (more favorable)

Okay	⟵	Caution
Caution	⟵	Danger

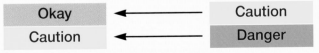

Occlusal risk factors for four teeth	Okay	Caution	Danger
WP WP RP	Highly unfavorable occlusal context		
WP WP WP	Favorable occlusal context	Moderately unfavorable occlusal context	Highly unfavorable occlusal context
RP RP RP RP	Highly unfavorable occlusal context		
RP RP RP	Moderately unfavorable occlusal context	Highly unfavorable occlusal context	
RP RP	Favorable occlusal context	Moderately unfavorable occlusal context	Highly unfavorable occlusal context

Occlusal risk factors for four teeth	Okay	Caution	Danger
	Moderately unfavorable occlusal context	Highly unfavorable occlusal context	
	Favorable occlusal context	Moderately unfavorable occlusal context	Highly unfavorable occlusal context
	Moderately unfavorable occlusal context	Highly unfavorable occlusal context	

Note

If the implants are placed offset from the center of the occlusal table, at the position of the buccal or lingual cusps, the recommendation is moved one step to the right (less favorable).

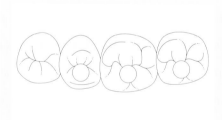

| Okay | ⟶ | Caution |
| Caution | ⟶ | Danger |

Note

If the implants are placed in a tripod configuration, the recommendation is moved one step to the left (more favorable).

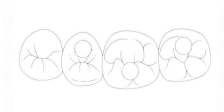

| Okay | ⟵ | Caution |
| Caution | ⟵ | Danger |

Note: This checklist is specific for the risk factors involved when three or four teeth are missing in the posterior maxilla. However, before an implant-supported restoration is planned for in this region, the general checklist should be utilized (see chapter 1, pages 14 and 15).

Maxilla: Complete-Arch Fixed Prostheses

Clinical situation *(Figs 4-79 and 4-80)*

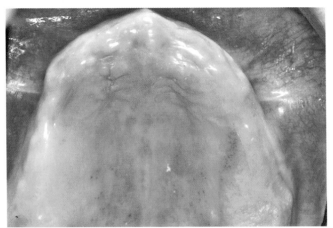

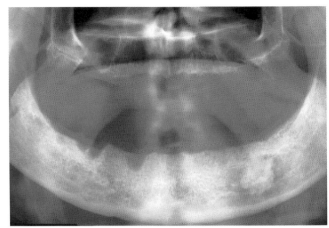

Fig 4-79   **Fig 4-80**

Conventional prosthetic solution

◼ Complete denture

Suggested implant solution *(Figs 4-81 to 4-85)*

Use of four to six implants, placed in an arch form, should be considered. In the posterior region, the 4-mm-diameter Regular Platform implant, or, if the bone volume allows, an even larger diameter implant should be used. It is important that the implants be spread in the anteroposterior direction. The restoration should be made on MirusCone abutments or standard abutments when considerable vertical bone resorption has taken place.

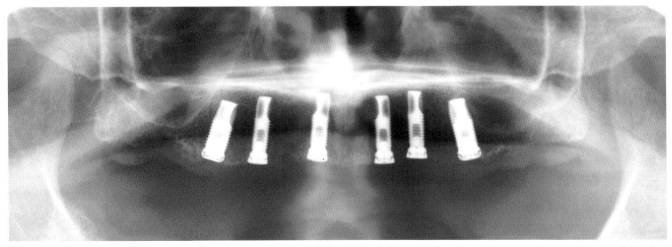

Fig 4-81 Six implants have been placed to treat a completely edentulous maxilla. Note the use of two Wide Platform implants posteriorly.

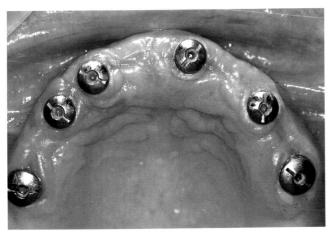

Fig 4-82 Same patient: Occlusal view during the placement of healing abutments. Note the spread of the implants along the crest.

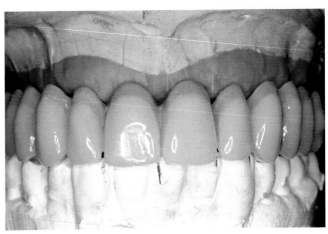

Fig 4-83 Complete-arch implant restoration. Note the height of the clinical crowns and their contact with the simulated gingiva. The minimal bone resorption has permitted the construction of a prosthesis with a "natural" dental profile. (Prosthesis by Dr J.-M. Gonzalez, Dr P. Rajzbaum, and C. Laval.)

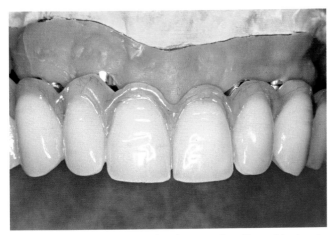

Fig 4-84 Complete-arch implant restoration. Moderate bone resorption has necessitated the realization of gingiva in rosy ceramic to mask the abutments and avoid phonetic problems. (Prosthesis by Dr J.-M. Gonzalez, Dr P. Rajzbaum, and C. Laval.)

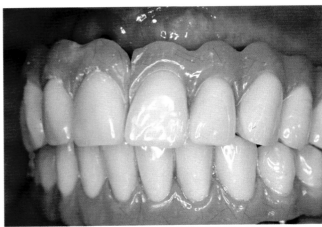

Fig 4-85 Two complete-arch dentures in the maxilla and the mandible. Major bone resorption has forced the fabrication of a large segment of false gingiva. Note the opening between the false gingiva and the mucosa to permit oral hygiene measures. (Prosthesis by Dr J.-M. Gonzalez, Dr P. Rajzbaum, and C. Laval.)

Alternative implant solution *(Figs 4-86 to 4-91)*

In patients with extreme bone resorption, or with a large maxillomandibular discrepancy, a prosthesis attached to a rigid bar should be considered. This type of construction makes it possible to place the implants in a more optimal position in accordance with the available bone volume and to benefit from the advantages of both the complete prosthesis (good lip support) and the fixed parial denture (lack of palatal contact). This solution also helps to solve phonetic problems and facilitates oral hygiene procedures.

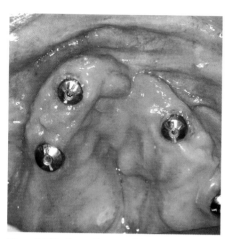

Fig 4-86 A patient with a labiopalatal cleft has been treated with a bone graft surgery. (Surgery by Dr P. Tessier.) The morphology of the crest does not permit the retention of a complete denture. Five implants have been placed in a manner to allow construction of a retention system for a prosthesis. One implant did not osseointegrate.

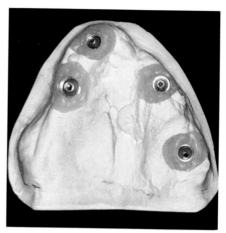

Fig 4-87 Same patient. Laboratory cast. A MirusCone abutment is placed on the Wide Platform implant in position 15. EsthetiCone abutments have been placed on the other implants.

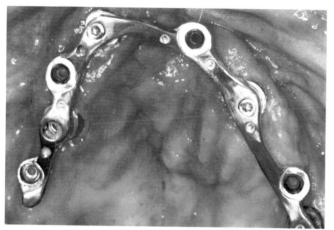

Fig 4-88 Same patient. A bar has been placed on the four implants. Note the four female parts of the attachments (Ceka).

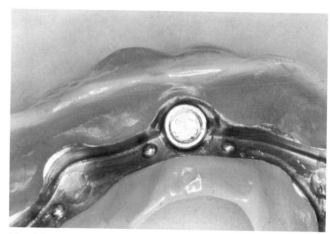

Fig 4-89 Same patient. Inside view of the prosthesis.

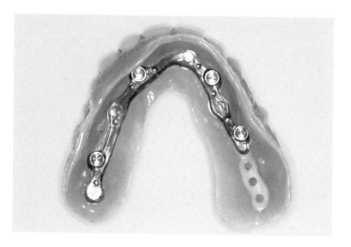

Fig 4-90 Same patient. Inside view of the prosthesis. Note the male parts of the attachments. A prosthetic palatal part is not necessary because of the good positioning of the implants and their adequate capacity to support the occlusal loads.

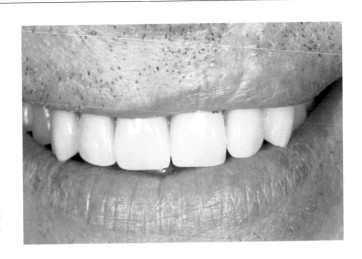

Fig 4-91 Same patient smiling, and with the prosthesis in place. (Prosthesis by Dr J.-M. Gonzalez, Dr P. Rajzbaum, X. Daniel, and P. Poussin.)

Limitations and risk factors

Limitation	Okay	Caution	Danger
Thickness of the osseous crest[1,2]	7 mm	6 mm	<5 mm
Height between osseous crest and opposing tooth[3]	7 mm	6 mm	<6 mm

[1] The dimensions given are for Regular Platform implants. If Wide Platform or 5-mm-diameter implants are used, 1 mm should be added.

[2] If the osseous crest is too thin, it is possible to enlarge it with bone regeneration or grafting techniques. In this situation, the healing time should be prolonged.

[3] The height should be measured from the level of osseous crest to the occlusal table of the opposing tooth.

Specific Risk Factors	Okay	Caution	Danger
Bone volume[1]	ABC	D	E
Bone density[2]	Type I-II-III	Type IV	
Number of implants	6	4	
Implant length	≥10 mm	6–8 mm	
Interimplant distance[3]	≥12 mm	≤8 mm	<4 mm
Occlusal context	Favorable	Unfavorable	Unfavorable + extension
Extension	None	1 tooth	2 teeth

[1] Bone volume after Lekholm and Zarb (1985).

[2] Bone density after Lekholm and Zarb (1985).

[3] Distance between implants measured as shown in Fig 5-56.

Technical note

It is possible to take an impression by using the surgical guide; this will allow transfer of the vertical interarch distance and the maxillomandibular relationship to the laboratory.

Maxilla: Implant-Supported Overdenture

Clinical situation *(Fig 4-92)*

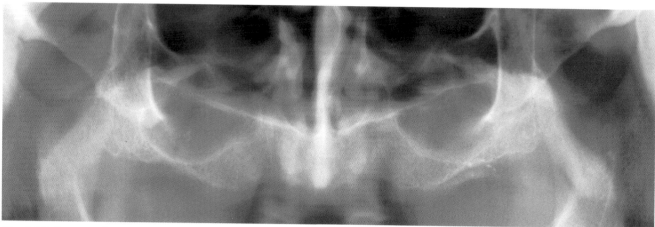

Fig 4-92 Panoramic radiograph. An implant solution is envisioned for the maxilla. The radiograph shows that the bone volume is insufficient for placement of implants behind the second premolars. An implant-supported overdenture is an interesting option for this kind of situation.

Conventional prosthetic solution

■ Complete denture

Suggested implant solution *(Figs 4-93 to 4-95)*

Use of four Regular Platform implants, in the positions of the lateral incisors and the first premolars, should be considered (if possible, 4 mm in diameter) on standard or MirusCone abutments.

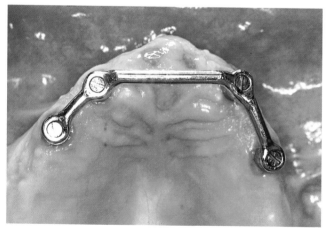

Fig 4-93 Four implants have been placed to support a bar. (Prosthesis by J. Ollier.)

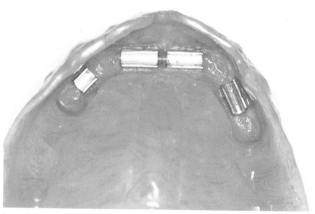

Fig 4-94 Same patient. Inside view of the prosthesis. Note the positions of the clips. (Prosthesis by Dr T. Nguyen and D. Raux.).

Note

This type of prosthesis may induce considerable forces on the implants and should not be considered a risk-free solution.

Note

Use of only two implants in this situation should be considered notably risky if the bone volume and density are not optimal.

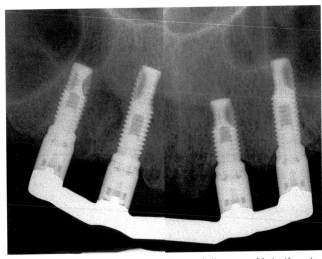

Fig 4-95 Same patient at the 3-year follow-up. Note the stable bone level around the implants.

Limitations and risk factors

Limitation	Okay	Caution	Danger
Interimplant distance	>10 mm	6–8 mm	<5 mm

Specific Risk Factors	Okay	Caution	Danger
Bone volume[1]	ABC	D	E
Bone density[2]	Type I-II-III	Type IV	
Implant length	>10 mm	6–8 mm	
Number of implants[3]	4–6	3–2	

[1] Bone volume after Lekholm and Zarb (1985)
[2] Bone density after Lekholm and Zarb (1985)
[3] Two implants should be considered extremely risky.

	Okay	This alternative represents the ideal solution. The clips should be placed between the implants to distribute the load.
	Okay	This solution is biomechanically less favorable than the previous solution because the lateral forces are less optimally distributed to all implants.
	Caution	
	Caution	This solution should be considered to represent a high biomechanical risk. The prosthesis should be considered as a fixed prosthesis supported by four implants with posterior extensions.
	Caution	This situation represents a moderate biomechanical risk. The implants could be overloaded by lateral forces. Note: It is important that implants be strictly parallel: prosthetic tolerance is less than 5 degrees.
	Danger	Use of only two implants should be considered an extreme biomechanical risk if the bone volume and quality are not optimal and/or if the patient presents with an unfavorable occlusal context.

Note: This checklist is specific for the risk factors involved with the implant-supported overdenture. However, before an implant-supported restoration is planned for in this region, the general checklist should be utilized (see chapter 1, pages 14 and 15).

Chapter 5

Treatment of the Edentulous Mandible

The preliminary examination makes it possible to identify risk patients and implant contraindications. After this analysis is made, the next step is to analyze the specific clinical situation based on the type of edentulism, because each type has its own requirements.

This chapter presents, type by type, proposed implant solutions and their specific limitations and risk factors.

In the tables, the limitations and risk factors are always presented in the same way:

	Okay	Caution	Danger
Risk factor or limitation	Ideal situation	Situation with moderate risk	Situation with major risk

The presence of several "cautions" represents a major risk situation and should lead to a reevaluation of the treatment plan.

If the risk factor is found in the "Danger" column, it is advised that the suggested implant solution be rejected.

Note: Occlusal context is explained in chapter 1, page 25.

Mandible: Central or Lateral Incisors

Clinical situation *(Fig 5-1)*

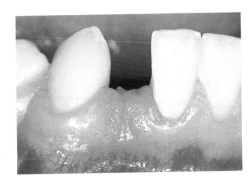

Fig 5-1 The patient has lost tooth 41 in a sports accident. The mesiodistal space is about 6 mm. An implant solution may be planned.

Conventional prosthetic solution

■ Resin-bonded prosthesis

Suggested implant solution *(Figs 5-2 to 5-5)*

Narrow Platform implant with the prosthetic restoration on an STR abutment.

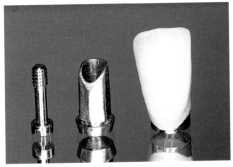

Fig 5-2 STR abutment with screw and ceramometal crown, replacing tooth 41.

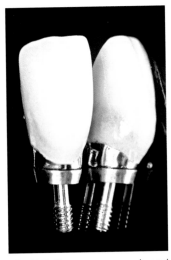

Fig 5-3 Same crown, placed on the abutment.

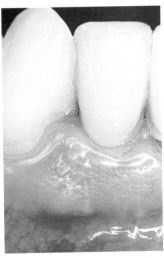

Fig 5-4 Patient with prosthesis, shown in Fig 5-3, in place. (Prosthesis by Dr E. Bouquet and M. Muller.)

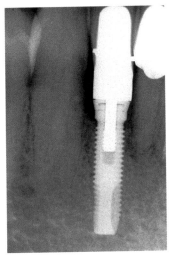

Fig 5-5 Same patient at follow-up 1 year after loading.

Note

Treatment of this type of edentulism is difficult and should be performed with a maximum of precautions. Generally, the mesiodistal space is too small for placing implants without the risk of touching the root of an adjacent tooth.

Limitations and risk factors

Limitation	Okay	Caution	Danger
Mesiodistal distance	6 mm	5 mm	<5 mm
Thickness of the osseous crest[1]	5 mm	4 mm	<4 mm
Height between the osseous crest and the opposing tooth[2]	7 mm	6 mm	<6 mm

[1] If the osseous crest is too thin, it is possible to enlarge it with bone regeneration or grafting techniques.
[2] The height should be measured from the level of osseous crest to the occlusal table of the opposing tooth. If a CeraOne abutment is used, the height must be a minimum of 7 mm.

Specific Risk Factors	Okay	Caution	Danger
Mucosal thickness	4–5 mm	<3 mm	
Vertical bone resorption[1]	None	Substantial	
Occlusal context	Favorable	Unfavorable	Unfavorable + offset

[1] The presence of a substantial vertical bone resorption is a health risk factor for the periodontal and peri-implant tissues. A discrepancy between the marginal bone level of the adjacent teeth and the level of the crest at the implant site represents a serious esthetic risk. Because of the proximity between teeth and implants, placement of the implants too deep relative to the line connecting the approximating cementoenamel junctions should be avoided (see Fig 1-19).

Note: This checklist is specific for the risk factors involved when the mandibular central or lateral incisor is missing. However, before an implant-supported restoration is planned for in this region, the general checklist should be utilized (see chapter 1, pages 14 and 15).

Mandible: Canine

Clinical situation *(Figs 5-6 and 5-7)*

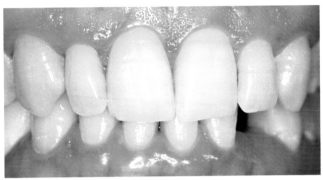

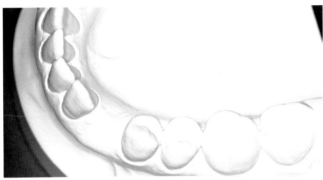

Fig 5-6 The patient has an ectopic tooth in position 33. It has not been possible orthodontically to replace the tooth in the arch. An implant solution is foreseen.

Fig 5-7 Same patient. Study case. The mesiodistal gap and the thickness of the crest are sufficient to allow implant placement.

Conventional prosthetic solution

- Fixed partial denture
- Resin-bonded prosthesis

Suggested implant solution *(Figs 5-8 and 5-9)*

Regular Platform implant, 4 mm in diameter, with a minimum length of 10 mm and the prosthetic restoration on a CeraOne abutment.

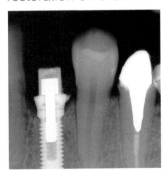

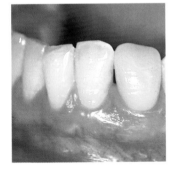

Fig 5-8 Same patient at placement of the CeraOne abutment.

Fig 5-9 Same patient. Final ceramometal crown. (Prosthesis by Dr J.-C. Furon, J. Dhont, and R. Standardi.)

Note

The implant should be placed in an ideal position in all three dimensions. If the implant axis is palatal to the incisal edge, a screw-retained prosthesis is viable. If the axis is buccal, a cemented-over solution should be considered (see page 69).

Key point

It is essential that a very precise surgical guide be used.

Alternative implant solution

If the implant position is not ideal in all three dimensions, or if the peri-implant mucosa is thin, presenting a risk of visibility, use of the TiAdapt or the CerAdapt abutment is recommended.

Note: To allow better adaptation of the prosthesis to the gingival contour, the TiAdapt or CerAdapt abutment may be indicated to improve the esthetic result.

Limitations and risk factors

Limitation	Okay	Caution	Danger
Mesiodistal distance	>7 mm	6 mm	<6 mm
Thickness of the osseous crest[1]	7 mm	5–6 mm	<4 mm
Height between the osseous crest and the opposing tooth[2]	7 mm	6 mm	<6 mm

[1] If the osseous crest is too thin, it is possible to enlarge it with bone regeneration or grafting techniques.

[2] The height should be measured from the level of osseous crest to the occlusal table of the opposing tooth. If a CeraOne abutment is used, the height must be a minimum of 7 mm.

Specific risk factors		Okay	Caution	Danger
Vertical bone resorption[1]		None	Substantial	
Mucosal thickness[2]		4–5 mm	<3 mm	
Implant diameter		4 mm	3.75 mm	3.3 mm
Occlusal context[3]	Regular Platform	Favorable	Unfavorable	Unfavorable + canine guidance
	Wide Platform	Unfavorable	Unfavorable + canine guidance	

[1] The presence of a substantial vertical bone resorption is a health risk factor for the periodontal and peri-implant tissues. A discrepancy between the marginal bone level of the adjacent teeth and the level of the crest at the implant site represents a serious esthetic risk.

[2] To obtain satisfactory peri-implant gingival morphology, tissue volume should be about 20% greater than the estimated need. This surplus allows the prosthodontist to adapt the gingiva to the prosthetic reconstruction.

[3] Because implants lack resilience, there is a risk of occlusal overload in the presence of canine guidance, and screw loosening may occur (see Alarm Signals, chapter 3). In a patient who exhibits bruxism or parafunction and canine guidance, use of a Wide Platform implant should be considered, if bone volume and bone density allow.

Note: This checklist is specific for the risk factors involved when the mandibular canine is missing. However, before an implant-supported restoration is planned for in this region, the general checklist should be utilized (see chapter 1, pages 14 and 15).

Technical note

It is possible to take an impression at the implant level during surgery. This makes it possible to attach a provisional crown at the second-stage surgery. The adaptation of the mucosa will be more precise.

Mandible: Premolar

Clinical situation *(Fig 5-10)*

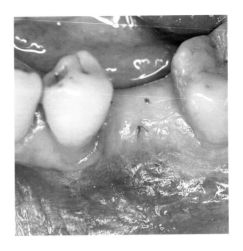

Fig 5-10 Tooth 35 has been extracted and should be replaced with an implant. The mesiodistal gap seems sufficient, and teeth 34 and 36 are intact.

Conventional prosthetic solution

- Fixed partial denture
- Resin-bonded prosthesis

Suggested implant solution *(Figs 5-11 and 5-12)*

Regular Platform implant, 4 mm in diameter, with a minimum length of 10 mm and the prosthetic restoration on a CeraOne abutment.

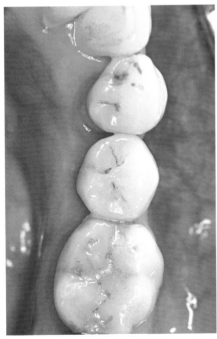

Fig 5-11 Same patient. Final prosthesis on a CeraOne abutment. (Prosthesis by Dr J.-C. Bonturi and P. Guillot.)

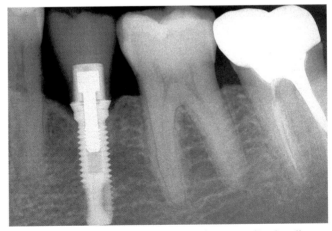

Fig 5-12 Same patient at follow-up 2 years after loading.

Alternative implant solution *(Figs 5-13 and 5-14)*

If the width of the bone crest allows (agenesis), the use of a Wide Platform implant is an alternative. For prosthetic reasons, the 5-mm-diameter Regular Platform implant could be considered.

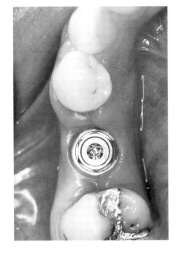

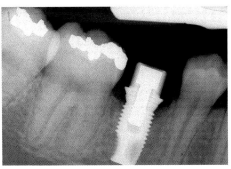

Fig 5-13 The patient has presented with agenesis at tooth 45. A Wide Platform implant has been used to acquire increased biomechanical strength for the prosthesis.

Fig 5-14 Same patient at placement of the CeraOne abutment.

Note

If the three-dimensional implant placement is not ideal, or if the peri-implant mucosa is thin, presenting a risk of abutment visibility, use of the CerAdapt abutment is recommended (Figs 5-15 to 5-18).

Fig 5-15 Tooth 35 should be replaced and tooth 36 should be restored.

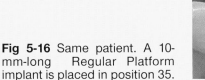

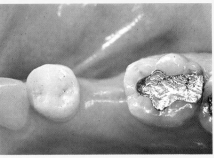

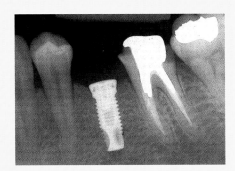

Fig 5-16 Same patient. A 10-mm-long Regular Platform implant is placed in position 35.

Fig 5-17 Same patient. CerAdapt abutment. The internal hexagon allows the use of the counter-torque device.

Fig 5-18 Same patient after placement of two In-Ceram crowns in positions 35 and 36. (Prosthesis by Dr J.-M. Gonzalez, Dr P. Rajzbaum, and N. Milliére.)

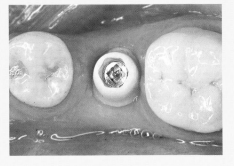

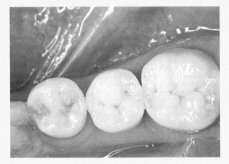

Limitations and risk factors

Limitation	Okay	Caution	Danger
Mesiodistal distance[1]	>7 mm	6 mm	<6 mm
Thickness of the osseous crest[2]	7 mm	6 mm	<5 mm
Height between the osseous crest and the opposing tooth[3]	7 mm	6 mm	<6 mm

[1] The dimensions given are for a Regular Platform implant. If a wider implant is used, 1 to 2 mm should be added.

[2] If the osseous crest is too thin, it is possible to enlarge it with bone regeneration or grafting techniques.

[3] The height should be measured from the level of osseous crest to the occlusal table of the opposing tooth. If a CeraOne abutment is used, the height must be a minimum of 7 mm.

Specific risk factors		Okay	Caution	Danger
Position of foramen[1]			Close to the crest	
Implant diameter		≥4 mm	3.75 mm	3.3 mm
Occlusal context[2]	Regular Platform	Favorable	Unfavorable	Unfavorable + lateral contacts
	Wide Platform	Unfavorable	Unfavorable + lateral contacts	

[1] Generally, the foramen is found between the premolars, slightly below the apices. The dental nerve bundle may loop in front of the foramen, which may put the nerve bundle at risk of being damaged during implant placement, leading to paresthesia or anesthesia of the lip. A computerized tomogram will effectively disclose such a nerve loop.

[2] Because implants are considerably more rigid than teeth, there is a risk that the implants may absorb a larger share of the load when mixed with natural teeth. Therefore, lateral occlusal contacts on the implant crown should be avoided and the cuspal inclination should be low.

Note: This checklist is specific for the risk factors involved when the mandibular premolar is missing. However, before an implant-supported restoration is planned for in this region, the general checklist should be utilized (see chapter 1, pages 14 and 15).

Technical note

It is possible to take an impression at the implant level during surgery. This makes it possible to place the definitive abutment and to attach a provisional crown at the second-stage surgery. The adaptation of the mucosa will be more precise.

Mandible: Molar

Clinical situation *(Fig 5-19)*

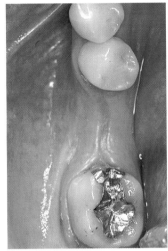

Conventional prosthetic solution

▨ Fixed partial denture

Fig 5-19

Suggested implant solution *(Figs 5-20 to 5-22)*

Wide platform implant with a minimum length of 10 mm and the prosthetic restoration on a CeraOne abutment.

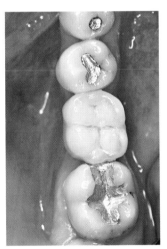

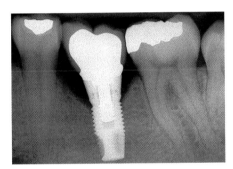

Fig 5-21 Same patient 6 months after loading. (The same case is presented in chapter 6, Figs 6-11 to 6-14.)

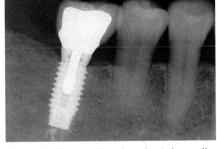

Fig 5-22 The patient is edentulous distal to tooth 45. From an occlusal viewpoint, a single tooth is sufficient. No functional risk factor has been found. A 5-mm-diameter Regular Platform implant is placed. Note the stability of the marginal bone after 3 years of function. (Prosthesis by Dr D. Vilbert and S. Tissier.)

Fig 5-20 The patient has lost tooth 46 to endodontic problems. The tooth has been replaced with a single crown cemented on a Wide Platform implant. (Prosthesis by Dr A. Foret-Duperier and N. Milliére.)

> **Note**
> The implant axis should be directed through the middle of the occlusal table to increase the biomechanical resistance of the restoration.

> **Note**
> When the bone in the posterior mandible is very dense, the use of a wide implant may lead to marginal bone resorption during the healing period. It seems preferable to avoid the use of Wide Platform implants in Type I bone.

Alternative implant solution *(Fig 5-23)*

If the mesiodistal space is wide (>12 mm), it is possible to use two Regular Platform implants to increase the biomechanical resistance of the restoration.

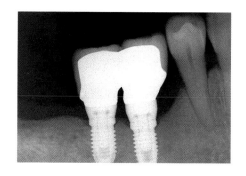

Fig 5-23 Radiograph at the 2-year follow-up. The patient is edentulous behind tooth 45. From an occlusal point of view, a single tooth is sufficient. However, the extensive vertical bone resorption necessitates placement of a high crown. To increase the biomechanical resistance of the system, it was decided to place two implants (8.5 and 7 mm long), rather than one Wide Platform implant 8.5 mm in length. (Prostheses by Dr G. Tirlet and S. Tissier.)

Limitations and risk factors

Limitation	Okay	Caution	Danger
Mesiodistal distance[1]	>8 mm	7 mm	<7 mm
Thickness of the osseous crest[2]	8 mm	6 mm	<5 mm
Height between the osseous crest and the opposing tooth[3]	7 mm	6 mm	<6 mm

[1] The dimensions given are for a Wide Platform implant. If a Regular Platform implant is used, 1 mm should be subtracted.
[2] If the osseous crest is too thin, it is possible to enlarge it with bone regeneration or grafting techniques.
[3] The height should be measured from the level of osseous crest to the occlusal table of the opposing tooth. If a CeraOne abutment is used, the height must be a minimum of 7 mm.

Specific Risk Factors	Okay	Caution	Danger
Nerve position		<8 mm from the crest	
Bone density[1]	Type I-II-III	Type IV	
Mesiodistal distance[2]	10 mm	>12 mm	
Implant length	10 mm	8.5 mm	<7 mm
Implant diameter	5 mm	4 mm	3.75 mm
Occlusal context[3]	Favorable	Unfavorable	Unfavorable + lateral contacts

[1] After a recent tooth extraction, the bone may have a low density. The use of large-diameter implants should, therefore, be considered. The healing time should be prolonged in Type IV bone.
[2] If the mesiodistal space is 12 mm or more, it is possible to place two Regular Platform implants.
[3] Implants are considerably more rigid than teeth; therefore, lateral occlusal contacts on the implant crown should be avoided and the cuspal inclination should be low.

Note: This checklist is specific for the risk factors involved when the mandibular molar is missing. However, before an implant-supported restoration is planned for in this region, the general checklist should be utilized (see chapter 1, pages 14 and 15).

Mandible: Anterior, Two Teeth Missing

Clinical situation *(Fig 5-24)*

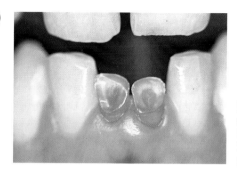

Fig 5-24 The patient presents with agenesis of teeth 31 and 41. Note the lack of available mesiodistal space. For this type of edentulism, an implant solution is rarely indicated.

Conventional prosthetic solution *(Fig 5-25)*

■ Resin-bonded prosthesis

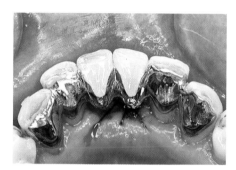

Fig 5-25 A resin-bonded prosthesis is used to replace teeth 31 and 41. Clinical situation after placement of the prosthesis. (Prosthesis by Dr J.-M. Gonzalez, Dr P. Rajzbaum, and C. Laval.)

Suggested implant solution *(Figs 5-26 to 5-30)*

Two Narrow or Regular Platform implants with single-crown restorations on CeraOne, TiAdapt, or CerAdapt abutments, or a splinted prosthesis on MirusCone or TiAdapt abutments.

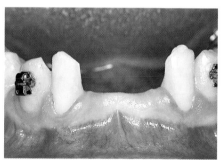 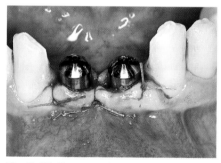

Fig 5-26 The patient presents with agenesis of teeth 31 and 41. To ensure a satisfactory anterior guidance, the implant solution has been requested by the orthodontist. The initial mesiodistal space was insufficient. Orthodontic correction has been made to allow the placement of two Narrow Platform implants. (Orthodontic treatment by Dr A. Fontenelle.)

Fig 5-27 Same patient at placement of the healing abutments. Because of the enlarged mesiodistal space, a prosthesis with three teeth is necessary.

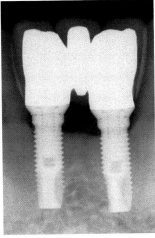

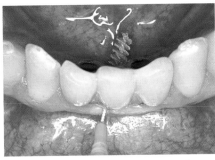

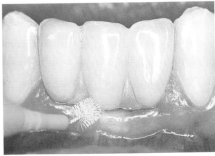

Fig 5-28 Same patient two years after loading. MirusCone abutments have been used.

Fig 5-29 Same patient at the 2-year follow-up.

Fig 5-30 Same patient at the 2-year follow-up. (Prosthesis by Dr Y. Samama and J. Ollier.)

Alternative implant solution *(Fig 5-31)*

If the mesiodistal space is insufficient for placement of two implants, it is possible to make two crowns on a 4-mm-diameter Regular Platform implant with a CeraOne or TiAdapt abutment.

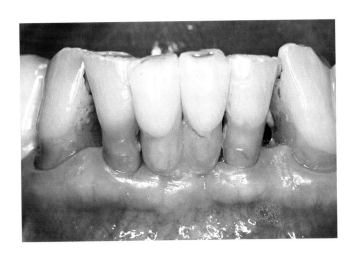

Fig 5-31 The patient is edentulous in positions 31 and 41. A single implant has been placed to support two crowns. Clinical view 2 years after loading. (The patient was treated by Dr H. Buisson. Reproduced with permission.)

Note

With this solution, the esthetics may be compromised and the biomechanical situation may be unfavorable.

Limitations and risk factors

Limitation	Okay	Caution	Danger
Mesiodistal distance (two implants)	>12 mm	10 mm	
Thickness of the osseous crest[1]	5 mm	4 mm	<4 mm
Height between the osseous crest and the opposing tooth[2]	7 mm	6 mm	<6 mm

[1] If the osseous crest is too thin, it is possible to enlarge it with bone regeneration or grafting techniques.

[2] The height should be measured from the level of osseous crest to the occlusal table of the opposing tooth. If a CeraOne abutment is used, the height must be a minimum of 7 mm.

Specific Risk Factors	Okay	Caution	Danger
Mucosal thickness[1]	4–5 mm	<3 mm	
Number of implants	2	1	
Occlusal context	Favorable	Unfavorable	Unfavorable + offset/cantilever

[1] To obtain satisfactory peri-implant gingival morphology, tissue volume should be about 20% greater than the estimated need. This surplus allows the prosthodontist to adapt the gingiva to the prosthetic reconstruction.

Note: This checklist is specific for the risk factors involved when two teeth are missing in the anterior mandible. However, before an implant-supported restoration is planned for in this region, the general checklist should be utilized (see chapter 1, pages 14 and 15).

Mandible: Anterior, Three or Four Teeth Missing

Clinical situation *(Fig 5-32 and 5-33)*

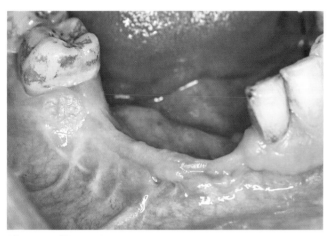

Fig 5-32 The patient has an ameloblastoma. The tumor is removed and the mandible is reconstructed with a bone graft. (Surgery by Dr Defresne.)

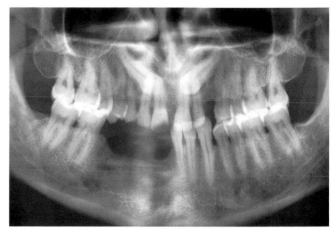

Fig 5-33 Same patient. Radiographic examination of the bone graft healing.

Conventional prosthetic solution

- Fixed partial denture
- Removable partial denture

Suggested implant solution *(Figs 5-34 to 5-36)*

Minimum of two Regular Platform implants and a prosthetic bridge on MirusCone or Standard abutments.

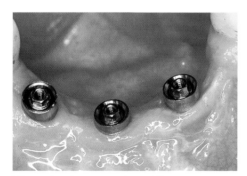

Fig 5-34 Same patient. Three implants have been placed in the bone graft. Standard abutments have been used.

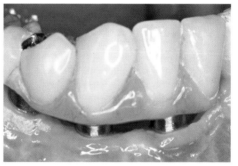

Fig 5-35 Same patient 3 years after loading of the prosthesis.

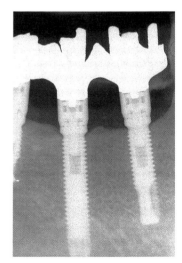

Fig 5-36 Same patient 3 years after loading. (Prosthesis by Dr J.-M. Gonzalez, Dr P. Rajzbaum, X. Daniel, P. Poussin.)

Attention

The Narrow Platform implant is 25% weaker than the 3.75-mm Regular Platform implant and should, therefore, be used for the replacement of a maximum of three teeth on two implants. If four teeth are replaced, it is recommended that Regular Platform implants be used, even if this could compromise the esthetics.

Alternative implant solution

Two Regular Platform implants with a prosthetic bridge on MirusCone abutments and one or two extensions.

Note

This solution should be considered to be associated with a moderate biomechanical risk.

Limitations and risk factors

Limitation	Okay	Caution	Danger
Thickness of the osseous crest[1]	5 mm	4 mm	<4 mm
Height between the osseous crest and the opposing tooth[2]	7 mm	6 mm	< 6 mm

[1] If the osseous crest is too thin, it is possible to enlarge it with bone regeneration or grafting techniques.
[2] The height should be measured from the level of osseous crest to the occlusal table of the opposing tooth.

Specific Risk Factors		Okay	Caution	Danger
Mucosal thickness[1]		4–5 mm	<3 mm	
Diameter of implants	Without extension	3.3 mm		
	With extension	3.75 mm	3.3 mm	
Occlusal context		Favorable	Unfavorable	Unfavorable + extension

[1] To obtain a satisfactory peri-implant gingival morphology, tissue volume should be about 20% greater than the estimated need. This surplus allows the prosthodontist to adapt the gingiva to the prosthetic reconstruction.

Note: This checklist is specific for the risk factors involved when three or four teeth are missing in the anterior mandible. However, before an implant-supported restoration is planned for in this region, the general checklist should be utilized (see chapter 1, pages 14 and 15).

Mandible: Posterior, Two Teeth Missing

Clinical situation *(Figs 5-37 and 5-38)*

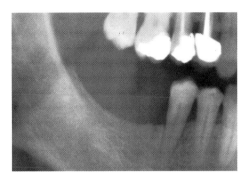

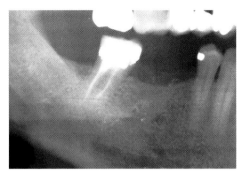

Fig 5-37 (Radiography by Dr G. Pasquet and Dr R. Cavezian.)

Fig 5-38 (Radiography by Dr G. Pasquet and Dr R. Cavezian.)

Conventional prosthetic solution

- Fixed partial denture
- Removable partial denture

Suggested implant solution

Missing Teeth	Implants
2 premolars (2 root supports)	2 Regular Platform 4 mm
1 premolar + 1 molar (3 root supports)	3 Regular Platform or 1 Regular + 1 Wide Platform
2 molars (4 root supports)	3 Regular Platform or 2 Wide Platform

When two teeth are missing between natural teeth, it is suggested that they be replaced by single-tooth abutments, CeraOne, or TiAdapt. The use of two splinted teeth on MirusCone or TiAdapt abutments is suggested for the free-end situation. Splinting is recommended in all situations in which the position or inclination of the implant axis is unfavorable.

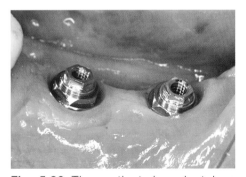

Fig 5-39 The patient is edentulous behind tooth 35. Wide Platform implants are placed in positions 36 and 37. Clinical view after placement of the MirusCone abutments.

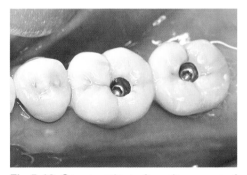

Fig 5-40 Same patient after placement of the screw-retained ceramometal prosthesis. Note the screw access holes. (Prosthesis by Dr J.-M. Gonzalez, Dr P. Rajzbaum, and N. Milliére.)

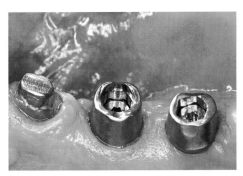

Fig 5-41 The patient is edentulous behind tooth 35. The occlusal context is favorable. Two implants have been placed in positions 36 and 37. Clinical situation at placement of the TiAdapt abutments. The internal hexagon allows the use of the countertorque device.

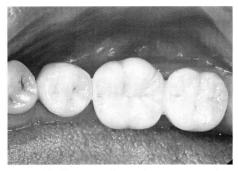

Fig 5-42 Same patient after cementation of the In-Ceram crowns. (Prostheses by Dr J.-M. Gonzalez, Dr P. Rajzbaum, and N. Milliére.)

Alternative implant solution

Sometimes, because of the position of the mental foramen, it is not possible to place the minimum of two implants for a free-end situation. When only a single implant can be placed posterior to the distal tooth, a prosthetic bridge may be made to connect to the implant to that tooth. Such a connection should be rigid to ensure that the occlusal forces are distributed equally between the implant and the tooth.

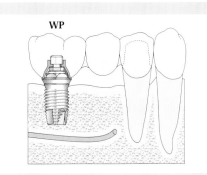

Fig 5-43

Note

This situation should be considered to entail a certain biomechanical risk (see the biomechanical checklist in chapter 3). If the bone volume and density allow, use of Wide Platform implants is recommended in this situation because of their larger load capacity (Fig 5-43).

Note

When the bone in the posterior mandible is very dense, the use of a wide implant may lead to marginal bone resorption during the healing period. It seems preferable to avoid the use of wide implants in Type I bone.

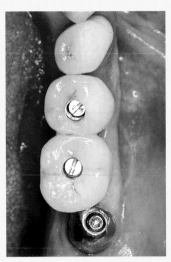

Note

If the occlusal context is unfavorable, three implants might be placed to increase support, even if only two teeth are necessary from an occlusal point of view (Figs 5-44 and 5-45).

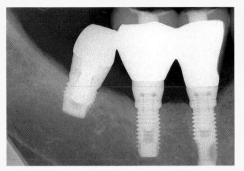

Fig 5-44 Teeth 45 and 46 have been replaced with an implant-supported prosthesis. Two teeth are necessary from a functional point of view. However, to strengthen the entire reconstruction, a supplementary implant has been placed distally.

Fig 5-45 Same patient at follow-up 2 years after loading. Note the stable peri-implant bone level. (Prosthesis by Dr G. Armandou and E. Davy.)

Limitations and risk factors

Limitation	Okay	Caution	Danger
Mesiodistal distance[1]	15 mm	<14 mm	
Thickness of the osseous crest[2]	7 mm	6 mm	<5 mm
Height between the osseous crest and the opposing tooth[3]	7 mm	6 mm	< 5 mm

[1] The dimensions given are for Regular Platform implants. If Wide Platform implants are used, 2 mm should be added.

[2] If the osseous crest is too thin, it is possible to enlarge it with bone regeneration or grafting techniques. In this situation, the healing time should be prolonged.

[3] The height should be measured from the level of osseous crest to the occlusal table of the opposing tooth. If a CeraOne abutment is used, the height must be a minimum of 7 mm.

Specific Risk Factors	Okay	Caution	Danger
Nerve position		<8 mm from the crest	
Implant diameter	≥4 mm	3.75 mm	3.3 mm
Occlusal context[1]	Favorable	Unfavorable	Unfavorable + extension

[1] Because implants are considerably more rigid than teeth, there is a risk that the implants may absorb a larger share of the load when mixed with natural teeth. Therefore, lateral occlusal contacts on the implant crown should be avoided, and the cuspal inclination should be low. It is especially important to eliminate lateral contacts for molar replacement, because the tooth most often is considerably larger than the implant platform.

Note: This checklist is specific for the risk factors involved when two teeth are missing in the posterior mandible. However, before an implant-supported restoration is planned for in this region, the general checklist should be utilized (see chapter 1, pages 14 and 15).

Mandible: Posterior, Three or Four Teeth Missing

Clinical situation
(Figs 5-46 and 5-47)

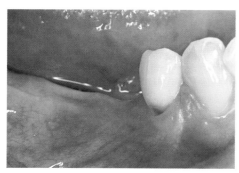

Fig 5-46 The patient is edentulous distal to tooth 44.

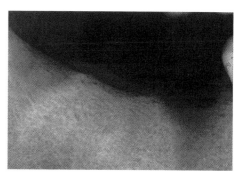

Fig 5-47 Same patient. Teeth 45 and 47 had been extracted 4 months earlier. The alveoli are visible on the radiograph. It is preferable to wait 2 to 3 months before placing the implants.

Conventional prosthetic solution

▓ Removable partial denture

Suggested implant solution *(Figs 5-48 and 5-49)*

Three Regular Platform implants, 4 mm in diameter, or Wide Platform implants with a bridge reconstruction on MirusCone abutments.

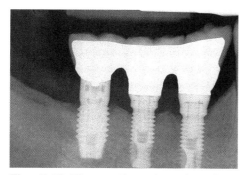

Fig 5-48 The patient is edentulous behind tooth 44. Three implants have been placed. Note the use of 5-mm-diameter Regular Platform implants in position 46. Note the stable bone margin after 3 years in function. (Prosthesis by Dr M. Bourdois and P. Lefauve.)

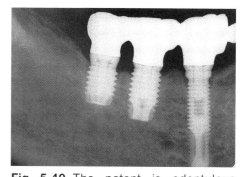

Fig 5-49 The patent is edentulous behind tooth 44. Three implants have been placed. Note the use of two 5-mm-diameter Regular Platform implants in teeth 45 and 46. Note the stable bone margin after 2 years in function. The prosthesis has been used as an orthodontic anchorage. (Orthodontic treatment by Dr A. Fontenelle.)

Note

When the bone in the posterior mandible is very dense, the use of a wide implant may lead to marginal bone resorption during the healing period. It seems preferable to avoid the use of wide implants in Type I bone.

Alternative implant solution

Sometimes only two implants can be placed. This situation is far from ideal and should be considered to entail a moderate to substantial biomechanical risk. In such situations, it is recommended that Wide Platform implants be used because of their larger load capacity.

> **Note**
> Connection of two implants with one or more natural teeth is not recommended. The splint can be considered as an unsupported extension to the implant prosthesis, because the implants have a much stiffer anchorage than the teeth. This situation represents a substantial biomechanical risk.

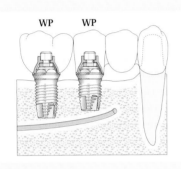

> **Note**
> If only two implants can be placed, it is preferable to connect only one to the teeth and to place a single crown on the other. The bending flexibility of the implant will compensate for the mobility of the tooth. Use of Wide Platform implants is recommended in this situation (Fig 5-50).

Fig 5-50

Limitations and risk factors

Limitation	Okay	Caution	Danger
Thickness of the osseous crest[1,2]	7 mm	6 mm	<5 mm
Height between the osseous crest and the opposing tooth[3]	7 mm	6 mm	<6 mm

[1] The dimensions given are for Regular Platform implants. If Wide Platform or 5-mm-diameter implants are used, 1 mm should be added.

[2] If the osseous crest is too thin, it is possible to enlarge it with bone regeneration or grafting techniques. In this situation, the healing time should be prolonged.

[3] The height should be measured from the level of osseous crest to the occlusal table of the opposing tooth. If a CeraOne abutment is used, the height must be a minimum of 7 mm.

Specific Risk Factors	Okay	Caution	Danger
Bone density	Type I-II-III	Type IV	
Nerve position		<8 mm from crest	
Number and positions of implants and occlusion (see table on next page)			

Occlusal risk factors for three teeth	Okay	Caution	Danger
RP RP RP	Moderately unfavorable occlusal context	Highly unfavorable occlusal context	
WP WP WP	Favorable occlusal context	Moderately unfavorable occlusal context	Highly unfavorable occlusal context
WP WP WP	Highly unfavorable occlusal context		
RP RP	Favorable occlusal context	Moderately unfavorable occlusal context	Highly unfavorable occlusal context
WP WP	Moderately unfavorable occlusal context	Highly unfavorable occlusal context	

Occlusal risk factors for three teeth	Okay	Caution	Danger
WP WP (see figure 5-50)	Moderately unfavorable occlusal context	Highly unfavorable occlusal context	
RP RP		Favorable occlusal context	Moderately unfavorable occlusal context
WP WP	Favorable occlusal context	Moderately unfavorable occlusal context	Highly unfavorable occlusal context

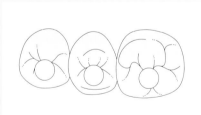

Note

If the implants are placed offset from the center of the occlusal table, at the position of the buccal or lingual cusps, the recommendation is moved one step to the right (less favorable).

Okay	⟶	Caution
Caution	⟶	Danger

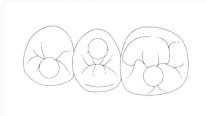

Note

If the implants are placed in a tripod configuration, the recommendation is moved one step to the left (more favorable).

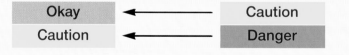

Okay	⟵	Caution
Caution	⟵	Danger

Occlusal factors for four teeth		Okay	Caution	Danger
WP WP WP		Highly unfavorable occlusal context		
RP RP RP RP		Highly unfavorable occlusal context		
WP WP RP		Favorable occlusal context	Moderately unfavorable occlusal context	Highly unfavorable occlusal context
RP RP RP		Moderately unfavorable occlusal context	Highly unfavorable occlusal context	
RP RP		Favorable occlusal context	Moderately unfavorable occlusal context	Highly unfavorable occlusal context

Occlusal factors for four teeth	Okay	Caution	Danger
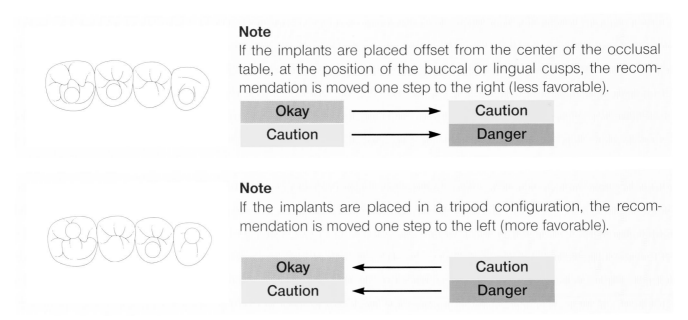	Moderately unfavorable occlusal context	Highly unfavorable occlusal context	
	Favorable occlusal context	Moderately unfavorable occlusal context	Highly unfavorable occlusal context
	Moderately unfavorable occlusal context	Highly unfavorable occlusal context	

Note

If the implants are placed offset from the center of the occlusal table, at the position of the buccal or lingual cusps, the recommendation is moved one step to the right (less favorable).

Okay	⟶	Caution
Caution	⟶	Danger

Note

If the implants are placed in a tripod configuration, the recommendation is moved one step to the left (more favorable).

Okay	⟵	Caution
Caution	⟵	Danger

Note: This checklist is specific for the risk factors involved when three or four teeth are missing in the posterior mandible. However, before an implant-supported restoration is planned for in this region, the general checklist should be utilized (see chapter 1, pages 14 and 15).

Mandible: Complete-Arch Fixed Prostheses

Clinical situation *(Figs 5-51 and 5-52)*

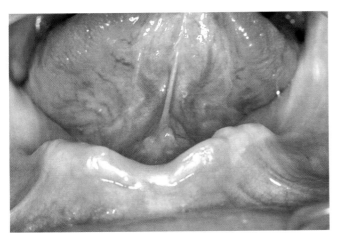

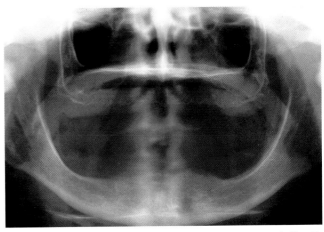

Fig 5-51 (Courtesy of Dr M. Pompignoli.)

Fig 5-52 (Radiography by Dr G. Pasquet and Dr R. Cavezian.)

Conventional prosthetic solution

■ Complete denture

Suggested implant solution *(Figs 5-53 to 5-55)*

Use of four to six implants placed in an arch form should be considered. In the posterior region, the 4-mm-diameter Regular Platform implant or, if the bone volume and bone density allow, even larger implants should be used. It is important that the implants be spread in the anteroposterior direction. The restoration should be made on MirusCone abutments or on standard abutments, when extensive vertical bone resorption has taken place.

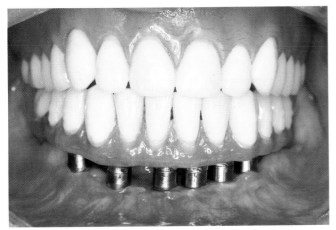

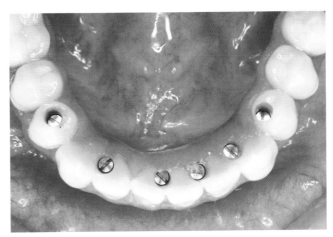

Fig 5-53 The patient is completely edentulous in both arches. The osseous crest in the mandible is severely resorbed. A prosthesis has been constructed on high abutment pillars. Situation 6 years after loading. (Prosthesis by Dr J.-M. Gonzalez, Dr P. Rajzbaum, and C. Laval.)

Fig 5-54 Same patient. Note the spread of the implants. Note the presence of two distal extensions.

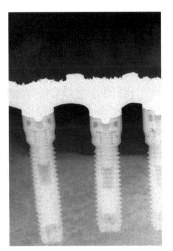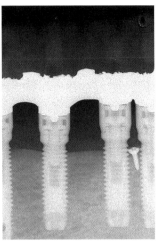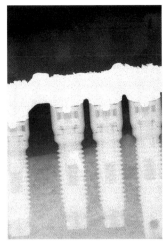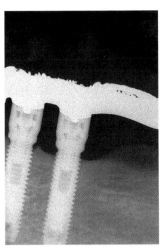

Fig 5-55 Same patient at the 6-year follow-up. Note the stable bone level around the implants. (For this patient, a bone regeneration technique was used. A membrane was fixed with microscrews. One screw had been left in place when the membrane was removed. Because of the total absence of any clinical symptoms, it was decided to leave the screw in place.)

Limitations and risk factors

Limitation	Okay	Caution	Danger
Thickness of the osseous crest[1,2]	7 mm	6 mm	<5 mm
Height between the osseous crest and the opposing tooth[3]	7 mm	6 mm	<6 mm

[1] The dimensions given are for Regular Platform implants. If Wide Platform and 5-mm-diameter implants are used, 1 mm should be added.

[2] If the osseous crest is too thin, it is possible to enlarge it with bone regeneration or grafting techniques. In this situation, the healing time should be prolonged.

[3] The height should be measured from the level of the osseous crest to the occlusal table of the opposing tooth.

Specific Risk factors	Okay	Caution	Danger
Bone volume[1]	ABC	D	E
Bone density[2]	Type I-II-III	Type IV	
Number of implants	6	4	
Implant length	≥10 mm	6–8 mm	
Interimplant distance[3]	>12 mm	<8 mm	<4 mm
Occlusal context[4]	Favorable	Unfavorable	Unfavorable + extension
Extension[4]	No	1 tooth	2 teeth

[1] Bone volume after Lekholm and Zarb (1985).
[2] Bone density after Lekholm and Zarb (1985).
[3] Distance between implants measured as shown in Fig 5-56.
[4] If the distance between the anterior and posterior implant is more than 8 mm, the suggestions may be shifted one step to the left in the table.

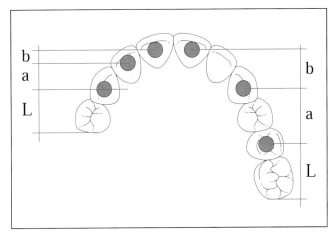

Fig 5-56

Note: This checklist is specific for the risk factors involved with complete-arch fixed prostheses in the mandible. However, before an implant- supported restoration is planned for in this region, the general checklist should be utilized (see chapter 1, pages 14 and 15).

Technical note
It is possible to take an impression by using the surgical guide; this will allow transfer of the vertical interarch distance to the laboratory.

Mandible: Implant-Supported Overdenture

Clinical situation *(Fig 5-57)*

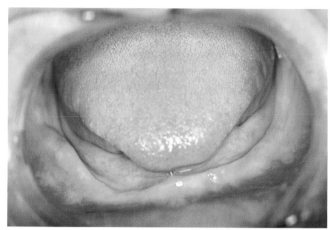

Fig 5-57

Conventional prosthetic solution

▨ Complete denture

Suggested implant solution

Two Regular Platform implants (4 mm in diameter, if possible) with standard or MirusCone abutments (for a bar design) (Figs 5-58 to 5-60) or Ball Attachment abutments (Fig 5-61).

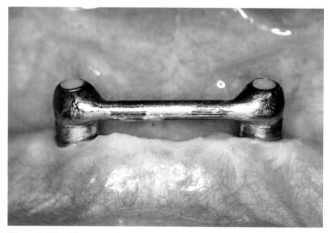

Fig 5-58 The patient has a completely edentulous mandible. Two implants have been placed in positions 33 and 43 to support a bar.

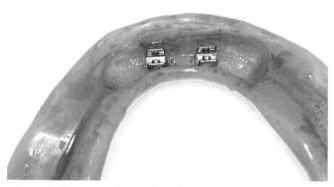

Fig 5-59 Same patient. View from underneath the prosthesis. Note the position of the clips.

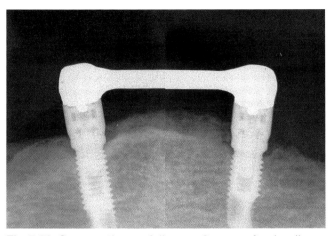

Fig 5-60 Same patient at follow-up 3 years after loading.

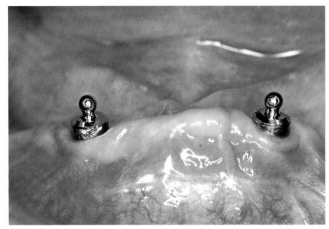

Fig 5-61 The patient has a completely edentulous mandible. Two implants have been placed in positions 33 and 43. Two abutments with ball attachments have been chosen. (Prosthesis by Dr P. Simonet.)

Note

The purpose of the implants is to improve the retention of the denture but not to support all forces during function. To reduce the load to the implants, the prosthetic support should be designed like a conventional prosthesis with respect to the support and stabilization criteria.

Limitations and risk factors

Limitation	Okay	Caution	Danger
Interimplant distance[1]	20 mm	<18 mm	

[1] To allow placement of two clips between the implants, the minimum distance should be 20 mm (Fig 5-62).

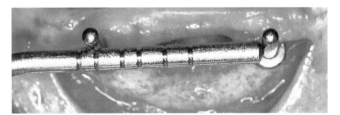

Figure 5-62

Specific risk factors	Okay	Caution	Danger
Number of implants[1]	2 or 4	3	
Implant length	>10 mm	<10 mm	

[1] Two implants provide a good geometry for the bar to act as a center of rotation for the prosthesis. Four implants may also be used for a support like that in a complete-arch fixed prosthesis. Three implants may lead to a less favorable situation, because the implant tripod might prevent the prosthesis from moving in response to occlusal forces.

Note: This checklist is specific for the risk factors involved with an implant-supported overdenture in the mandible. However, before an implant-supported restoration is planned for in this region, the general checklist should be utilized (see chapter 1, pages 14 and 15).

	Okay	This alternative represents the ideal solution. The bar should be oriented so that it allows a certain rotation of the prosthesis.
	Okay	This alternative also represents a reliable solution.
	Attention	This solution represents a substantial biomechanical risk. There is a risk of fracture of the extension and the implant components.
	Attention	This solution represents a major biomechanical risk, because the prosthesis cannot rotate. The implants will support all the load, and the solution should be considered to be a fixed prosthesis on three implants.
	Okay	This solution may function as a fixed prosthesis and has little biomechanical risk if the implants are well spread. Note: If ball attachments are used, implants must be strictly parallel. The prosthetic tolerance is less than 5 degrees. A bar solution is preferable.

Suggested Readings

Single-tooth edentulism

Andersson Ödman P, Boss A, Jörneus L. Mechanical testing of superstructures on the CeraOne abutment in the Brånemark System. Int J Oral Maxillofac Implants 1994;9:665-672.

Balshi TJ, Hernadez RE, Pryszlak MC, Rangert B. A comparative study of one implant versus two replacing a single molar. Int J Oral Maxillofac Implants 1996;11:372-378.

Balshi TJ, Wolfinger GJ. Two-implant-supported single molar replacement: Interdental space requirements and comparison to alternative options. Int J Periodont Rest Dent 1997;17:427-435.

Becker W, Becker B. Replacement of maxillary and mandibulary molars with single endosseous implant restorations: A retrospective study. J Prosthet Dent 1995;74:51-55.

Henry P, Laney W, Jemt T, Harris D, Krogh P, Polizzi G, Zarb G, Herrmann I. Osseointegrated implants for single-tooth replacement: A prospective multicenter study. Int J Oral Maxillofac Implants 1996;11:450-455.

Jemt T, Lekholm U, Grondahl. A 3-year follow-up study of early single implant restorations ad modum Brånemark. Int J Periodont Rest Dent 1990;10:341-349.

Laney W, Jemt T, Harris D, Henry P, Krogh P, Polizzi G, Zarb G, Herrmann I. Osseointegrated implants for single-tooth replacement: Progress report from a multicenter prospective study after 3 years. Int J Oral Maxillofac Implants 1994;9:49-54.

Pestipino V, Ingber A, Kravitz J. Clinical and laboratory considerations in the use of a new all-ceramic restorative system. Pract Periodont Aesthet Dent 1998;10:567-575.

Partial edentulism

Higuchi K, Folmer T, Kultje C. Implant survival rates in partially edentulous patients. A 3-year prospective multicenter study. J Oral Maxillofac Surg 1995;53:264-268.

Jemt T, Lekholm U. Oral implant treatment in the posterior partially edentulous jaw: A 5-year follow-up report. Int J Oral Maxillofac Implants 1993;8:635-640.

Lekholm U, van Steenberghe D, Herrmann I, Bolender C, Folmer T, Gunne J, Henry P, et al. Osseointegrated implants in the treatment of partially edentulous jaws: A prospective 5-year multicenter study. Int J Oral Maxillofac Implants 1994;9:627-635.

Naert J, Quirynen H, van Steenberghe D, Darius P. A six-year prosthodontic study of 509 consecutively inserted implants for the treatment of partial edentition. J Prosthet Dent 1992;67:236-245.

Nevins M, Langer B. The successful application of osseointegrated implants to the posterior jaw: A long-term retrospective study. Int J Oral Maxillofac Implants 1993;8:428-432.

Tulasne JF. Implant treatment of missing posterior dentition. In: Albrektsson T, Zarb GA (eds). The Brånemark Osseointegrated Implants. Chicago: Quintessence, 1988.

Complete edentulism

Adell R, Eriksson B, Lekholm U, Brånemark P-I, Jemt T. A long-term follow-up study of osseointegrated implants in the treatment of totally edentulous jaw. Int J Oral Maxillofac Implants 1990;5:347-359.

Adell R, Lekholm U, Rockler B, Brånemark P-I. A 15-year study of osseointegrated implants in the treatment of the edentulous jaw. Int J Oral Surg 1981;10:387-416.

Brånemark P-I, Hansson B, Adell R, Breine U, Lindström J, Hallén O, Öhman A. Osseointegrated implants in the treatment of the edentulous jaw. Experience from a 10-year period. Stockholm: Almqvist and Wiksell International, 1977

Jemt T, Lekholm U. Implant treatment in edentulous maxillae: A 5-year follow-up report on patients with different degrees of jaw resorption. Int J Oral Maxillofac Implants 1995;10:303-311.

Lundqvist S, Haraldson T, Lindblad P. Speech in connection with maxillary fixed prostheses on osseointegrated implants: A three-year follow-up study. Clin Oral Implants Res 1992;3:176-180.

Lundqvist S, Lohmander-Agerskov A, Haraldson T. Speech before and after treatment with bridges on osseointegrated implants in the edentulous. Clin Oral Implants Res 1992;3:57-62.

Tolman D, Laney R. Tissue-integrated prosthesis complications. Int J Oral Maxillofac Implants 1992;7:477-484.

Zarb G, Schmitt A. The longitudinal clinical effectiveness of osseointegrated dental implants. Part III. Problems and complications encountered. J Prosthet Dent 1990;64:185-194.

Overdenture

Hutton JE, Heath R, Chai JY, et al. Factors related to success and failure rates at 3-year follow-up in a multicenter study of overdentures supported by Brånemark implants. Int J Oral Maxillofac Implants 1995;10:33-42.

Jemt T, Chai J, Harnett J, et al. A 5-year prospective multicenter follow-up report on overdentures supported by osseointegrated implants. Int J Oral Maxillofac Implants 1996;11:291-298.

Petropoulos VC, Woollcott S, Kousvelari E. Comparison of retention and release periods for implant overdenture attachments. Int J Oral Maxillofac Implants 1997;12:176-185.

Naert I, Quirynen M, Theuniers G, van Steenberghe D. Prosthetic aspect of osseointegrated fixtures supporting overdentures. A 4-year report. J Prosthet Dent 1991;65:671-680.

Implants connected to natural teeth

Åstrand P, Borg K, Gunne J, Olsson M. Combination of natural teeth and osseointegrated implants as prosthesis abutments. A 2-year longitudinal study. Int J Oral Maxillofac Implants 1991;6:305-312.

Gunne J, Åstrand P, Ahlén K, Borg K, Olsson M. Implants in partially edentulous patients. A longitudinal study of bridges supported by both implants and natural teeth. Clin Oral Implants Res 1993;3:49-56.

Olsson M, Gunne J, Åstrand P, Borg K. Free-standing implant-supported bridges versus tooth-implants-supported bridges: A five-year prospective study. Clin Oral Implants Res 1995;6:114-121.

Wide diameter implants

Langer B, Langer L, Herrmann I, Jörnéus L. The wide fixture: A solution for special bone situations and a rescue for a compromised implant. Part 1. Int J Oral Maxillofac Implants 1993;8:400-408.

Impression at implant level

Kupeyan HK, Brien RL. The role of the implant impression in abutment selection: A technical note. Int J Oral Maxillofac Implants 1995;10:429-433.

Prestipino V, Ingber A. Implant fixture position registration at the time of fixture placement surgery. Pract Periodont Aesthet Dent 1992;5:1-7.

Resin-bonded prostheses

Samama Y. Fixed bonded prosthodontics: A 10-year follow-up report. Part I. Analytical overview. Int J Periodont Rest Dent 1995;5:425-435.

Samama Y. Fixed bonded prosthodontics: A 10-year follow-up report. Part II. Clinical assessment. Int J Periodont Rest Dent 1996;16:53-59.

Screw-retained versus cemented prostheses

Ingber A, Prestipino V. Differentiating between the use of cemented and screw-retained prostheses on root-form implants. Dent Implantol Update 1994;5:33-37.

Hebel K, Gajjar RC. Cement-retained versus screw-retained implant restorations: Achieving optimal occlusion and esthetics in implant dentistry. J Prosthet Dent 1997;77:28-35.

Additional readings

Engleman MJ. Clinical Decision Making and Treatment Planning in Osseointegration. Chicago: Quintessence, 1997.

Hobo S, Ichida E, Garcia LT. Osseointegration and Occlusal Rehabilitation. Chicago: Quintessence, 1990.

Nevins M, Mellonig JT. Implant Therapy: Clinical Approaches and Evidence of Success, vol 2. Chicago: Quintessence, 1998.

Palacci P, Ericsson I, Engstrand P, Rangert B. Optimal Implant Positioning and Soft Tissue Management for the Brånemark System. Chicago: Quintessence, 1995.

Parel SM. The Smiline System. Dallas, TX: Stephen M. Parel, 1991.

Parel SM, Sullivan DY. Esthetics and Osseointegration. Dallas, TX: Osseointegration Seminars, 1989.

Strub JR, Witkowski S, Einsele F. Prosthodontic aspect of implantology. In Watzek G (ed). Endosseous Implants: Scientific and Clinical Aspects. Chicago: Quintessence, 1996.

Treatment Sequence and Planning Protocol

The established treatment sequence and planning protocol allows a high and predictable success rate. The surgical sequence and the different phases of healing and loading have been defined since the late 1960s. However, clinical experience and documentation have demonstrated that there is room for modification of the original protocol for the individual clinical situation, regarding both sequence and technique.

Implant treatment in general follows the schedule indicated below:

Clinical examination: General and specific indications and contraindications (see chapters 1 to 3)

Radiographic examination: surgical indications and contraindications

Fabrication of a surgical guide: prosthetic demands

Surgical and prosthetic phases

Maintenance phase

Radiographic Examination

The radiographic examination is indispensable for determining the volume and density of the bone.

Bone volume

It is important to distinguish among available bone volume, necessary bone volume, and useful bone volume.

The available volume represents the total amount of bone in which it is theoretically possible to place an implant in a certain region. This may be evaluated by means of a computerized tomographic scanner or a Scanora. The information does not consider the prosthodontic parameters but rather is a strict surgical evaluation.

The necessary volume represents the minimum amount of bone required for placement of an implant that will function in the given clinical situation. This is not an anatomic parameter of the patient but rather a theoretical value. It may be defined by using the checklists for limitations and risks factors (see chapters 4 and 5).

Example for single-molar replacement

Limitation	Okay	Caution	Danger
Mesiodistal distance	>8 mm	7 mm	<7 mm
Width of osseous crest	8 mm	6 mm	<5 mm
Height between the osseous crest and the opposing tooth	7 mm	6 mm	<6 mm

Specific Risk Factors	Okay	Caution	Danger
Position of sinus		Base	
Bone density	Type I-II-III	Type IV	
Mesiodistal distance	10 mm	<12 mm	
Implant length	10 mm	8.5 mm	<7 mm
Implant diameter	5 mm	4 mm	3.75 mm
Occlusal context	Favorable	Unfavorable	Unfavorable lateral contact

The necessary bone volume for this type of restoration is ideally a minimum of 8 × 8 × 10 mm.

The useful volume represents the amount of bone that can be utilized in a given clinical situation, considering the prosthodontic parameters (esthetic as well as functional). It can objectively be specified preoperatively with a CT scan or a Scanora, by using a guide with radiographic markers (discussed later). If the useful volume is much less than the necessary volume, the implant treatment plan should be reevaluated

Bone augmentation techniques (see below) could be investigated in order to increase the amount of useful bone.

Note
If only the available bone volume is considered during the preoperative examination, the prosthetic result may suffer.

Summary (Fig 6-1)
Available volume = surgical evaluation
Necessary volume = prosthetic evaluation
Useful volume   = surgical + prosthetic evaluation

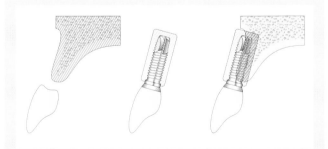

Fig 6-1 Available bone volume (green), necessary bone volume (blue), and useful bone volume (red).

Bone Density

Bone density is a difficult parameter to evaluate. It varies substantially from one anatomic region to another and may even vary considerably within the same operating zone. However, the knowledge of bone density is extremely important to establishment of the treatment plan. The failure rate is greater for regions with very low density (low primary stability) or regions with very high density (risk for overheating during drilling).

A good evaluation of bone density allows the surgeon to do the following:

- Select the proper implant diameter
- Decide about the optimal drilling sequence (in soft bone: use of final drill to half depth only, minimal use of countersink, use of smaller drill diameters than standard, etc; in hard bone: use of oversized drill diameters).
- Determine the length of the healing period.
- Evaluate the occlusal load capacity of the different implants.

Classification of bone quality

Bone quality can be evaluated with two parameters. The first (Types I, II, III, and IV) according to Lekholm and Zarb (1985), classifies the bone quality from a mechanical aspect (bone density); the second parameter classifies bone from a healing standpoint (bone biology).

Classification of bone density (Lekholm and Zarb, 1985) *(Figs 6-2 to 6-5)*

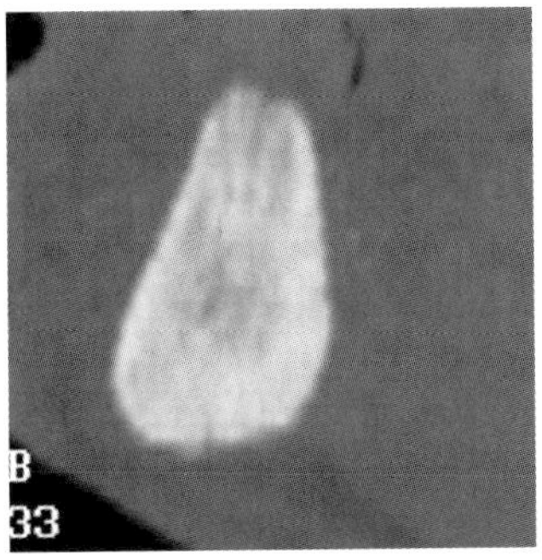

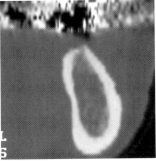

Fig 6-2 Radiograph of a mandible: The bone is very dense and homogenous: Type I bone. (Radiography by Dr N. Bellaïche.)

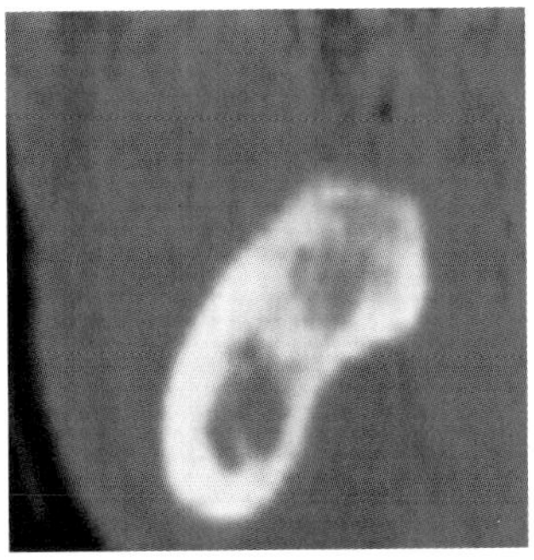

Fig 6-3 Radiograph of a mandible: The cortex is very thin and the cancellous bone appears dense. Type II bone. (Radiography by Dr N. Bellaïche.)

Fig 6-4 Radiograph of a mandible: The cortex is fine and the cancellous bone appears sparse. Type III bone. (Radiography by Dr N. Bellaïche.)

Fig 6-5 Radiograph of a mandible: The cortex is not visible and the medullar bone appears very sparse. Type IV bone. (Radiography by Dr N. Bellaïche.)

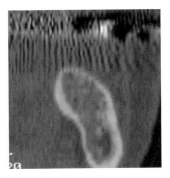

Certain habits (eg, smoking), disease (eg, osteoporosis), or medication (corticosteroid) may modify the healing capacity of the bone. A classification is suggested for dividing the bone-healing potential (BHP) into three categories: BHP 1, 2, and 3.

Note

Type II bone (high density) in a heavy smoker may well have a low healing potential (BHP 3). This patient should be considered a risk patient, even if the bone density evaluated on radiographs is satisfactory.

Density

Type I:	Essentially cortical bone
Type II:	Dense corticocancellous bone
Type III:	Sparse corticocancellous bone
Type IV:	Thin cortical and very sparse medullar bone

Quality

BHP 1:	Bone with normal healing potential
BHP 2:	Bone with moderately reduced healing potential
	Possible reasons:
	Moderate smoking (approximately 10 cigarettes a day)
	Controlled diabetes
	Osteoporosis
	Nutrition deficiency
	Bone graft
	Regenerated bone
	Long-term treatment with corticosteroids
	Long-term treatment with nonsteroidal anti-inflammatory agents (indomethacin)
BHP 3:	Bone with a substantially reduced healing potential
	Possible reasons:
	Heavy smoking (20 or more cigarettes a day)
	Hyperparathyroidism
	Thalassemia
	Gaucher's disease
	Paget's disease
	Fibrous dysplasia
	Diabetes mellitus
	Severe anemia
	Antimitotic treatment
	Severe osteoporosis
	Irradiated bone
	Rheumatoid arthritis

Surgical risk factors associated with bone density and quality

	Type I	Type II	Type III	Type IV
BHP 1:	Okay	Okay	Okay	Caution
BHP 2:	Caution	Okay	Okay	Caution/Danger
BHP 3:	Caution	Caution	Caution	Danger

Okay = Standard surgical protocol
Caution = Very gentle surgical technique, rigorous aseptic protocol, prolonged healing time. No pressure from the provisional prosthesis during healing.
Danger = A patient with a severe risk should only be treated by a highly experienced team.

A precise bone evaluation is difficult to perform in daily practice, because means are lacking for an exact analysis. Still, there are many ways of determining the bone density.

Radiographic evaluation *(Figs 6-6 and 6-7)*

Radiographic evaluation is the simplest and most commonly used technique but not always the most sensitive.

Advantages
- Simple.
- Sensitive enough for medium densities.

Disadvantages
- Difficult to interpret in extreme situations.
- Does not take into account that the implant does not necessarily fall into one radiographic section.

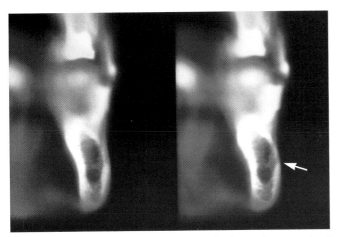

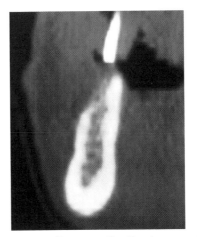

Fig 6-6 Preoperative Scanora view before placement of implants in the mandibular left segment. The radiographic image covers the area to the mental foramina *(arrow)*. The contour of the mandible is very distinct. The cortex is thick. The cancellous bone seems to have a high density. This mandible, at the level of this radiograph, has a density of Type II. (Radiography by Dr G. Pasquet and Dr R. Cavezian.)

Fig 6-7 Preoperative Dentascan of proposed implant sites in the mandibular right segment. The section of the image passes just behind the mental foramina. Note the radiographic markers in the surgical guide. The crestal cortex is fine and partly absent; the cancellous bone appears dense. This mandible, at the level of this image, has a density of Type III. (Radiography by Dr M. Giwerc.)

Computer tomographic evaluation *(Fig 6-8)*

Radiographs are available as conventional films but also as digital information on diskettes, which allows the practitioner to make the examination on a personal computer. With the latter option, it is possible to evaluate the bone density with specific computer programs.

Advantages
● Provides clinically reliable preoperative examination.
● Allows assessment of bone density in any possible direction of implant placement.

Disadvantages
● Requires a computer with an appropriate program.
● Increases the total treatment cost.

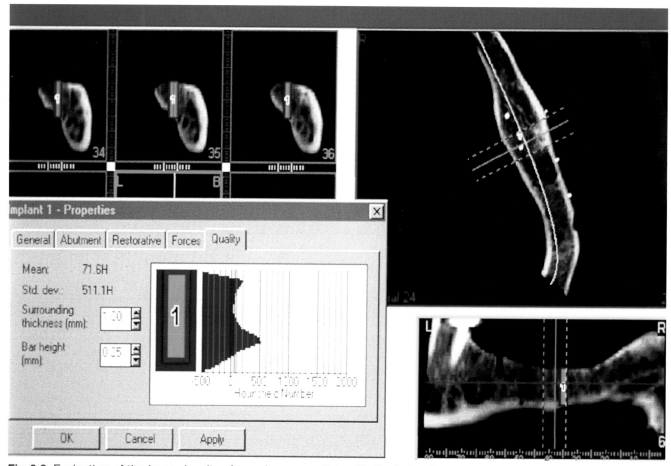

Fig 6-8 Evaluation of the bone density of a cadaver mandible with the help of a computer. Photograph of the computer screen during use of the Simplant program. (Radiography by Dr N. Bellaïche.) A virtual implant is placed on the scanner images. The computer program calculates the bone density around the implant and displays the evaluation in the form of a graph. This graph represents the bone density value along the implant axis.

Evaluation by drilling and tapping resistance *(Figs 6-9 to 6-14)*

It is possible to measure the torque resistance during use of a screw tap or placement of the implant. The OsseoCare DEC 600 drilling equipment has a display that shows the resistance versus the time. The graph represents a measure of the implant stability.

From these curves, it may be possible to determine the required healing time for each implant. It would also be possible to use the graphs to indicate if one-stage surgery or immediate loading protocols could be applied.

Advantage
● Provides a good evaluation of the clinically achieved implant stability.

Disadvantages
● Is sometimes difficult to interpret.
● Provides only a retrospective evaluation.

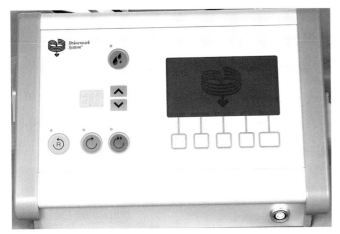

Fig 6-9 DEC 600 drilling unit. The tapping resistance at low speed is registered and displayed on the screen as a graph.

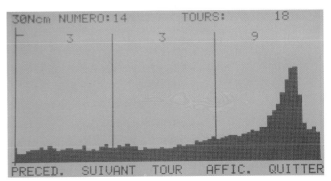

Fig 6-10 Graph obtained during tapping resistance measurement with DEC 600. The registration is done during implant placement. The site is drilled at the same position as the virtual implant in Fig 6-8. The graph corresponds to the tapping resistance versus time. The decrease of the resistance in the graph at the end of the operation corresponds to the perforation of the cortex by the implant. This is shown as a reduction of the radiographic density as well as tapping resistance.

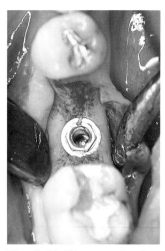

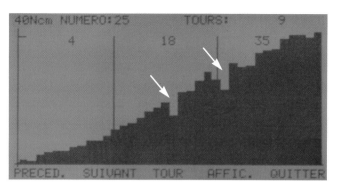

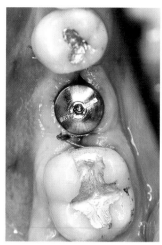

Fig 6-11 Placement of a Wide Platform implant in position 46.

Fig 6-12 Same patient. The tapping resistance was registered during implant placement. Placement of the implant commenced at 20 N/cm and the motor stopped *(left arrow)*. The torque was increased to 30 N/cm and then the motor stopped again *(right arrow)*. The final placement was at 40 N/cm. The graph demonstrates perfect initial stability of the implant at the end of the placement procedure.

Fig 6-13 Same patient. Favorable situation associated with the perfect initial stability of the implant allows for a one-stage surgical technique. The healing abutment is placed on the implant. The mucosal flaps are sutured face to face.

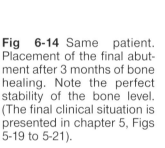

Fig 6-14 Same patient. Placement of the final abutment after 3 months of bone healing. Note the perfect stability of the bone level. (The final clinical situation is presented in chapter 5, Figs 5-19 to 5-21).

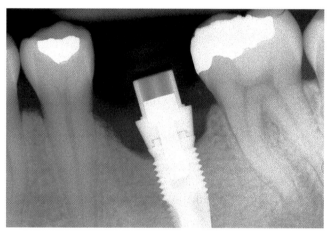

Preliminary Radiographic Examination

Panoramic radiograph. This is an indispensable radiographic examination (Fig 6-15). It provides a total view of the situation, allows an approximate measurement of the bone volume, and makes it possible to detect in advance contraindications arising from too little bone volume.

Retroalveolar radiograph. This view refines the diagnostic investigation in particular situations, such as evaluation of the distance between roots (eg, for replacement of a maxillary lateral incisor), examination for interdental bone peaks (see chapter 2), and evaluation of vertical bone resorption (see chapter 2) (Fig 6-16).

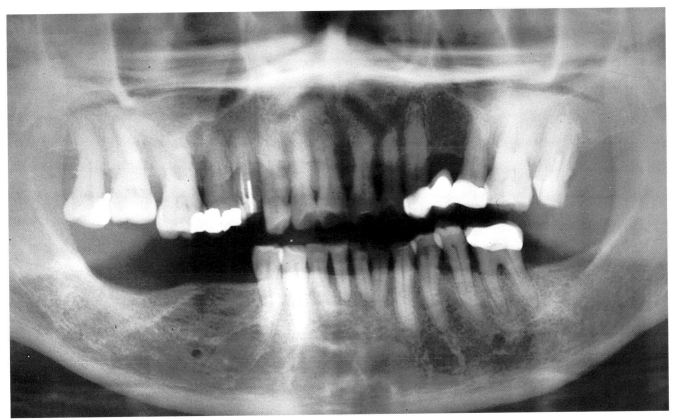

Fig 6-15 Preoperative panoramic radiograph. Implants are to be placed in the mandibular left and right segments. The radiographic analysis reveals that in the right segment it is possible to insert an implant in front of the mental foramina and that the available bone height above the inferior alveolar nerve seems sufficient. However, for a precise evaluation of the available bone volume, it is necessary to complement the radiographic investigation with a three-dimensional presentation by means of a scanner or Scanora. (Radiography by Dr G. Pasquet and Dr R. Cavezian.)

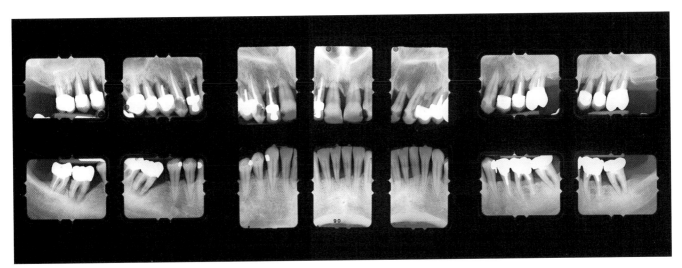

Fig 6-16 Radiographic status.

Preoperative Radiographic Examination

The Scanora gives a tomographic representation. The radiologist delivers both a panoramic view (1.3 enlargement) and cross sections (1.7 enlargement). The Scanora is a simple and reliable examination but sometimes difficult to evaluate (Figs 6-17 and 6-18).

Computerized tomographic scanning is a tomographic density examination that delivers axial (horizontal) or frontal (vertical) sections. Special computer programs have been developed for preimplant evaluation. Based on the axial sections, the program reconstructs the sagittal sections perpendicular to the osseous crest. The images are presented in a natural scale (1:1). The interpretation of these images is simple, but the cost to produce them is relatively high (Figs 6-19 and 6-20).

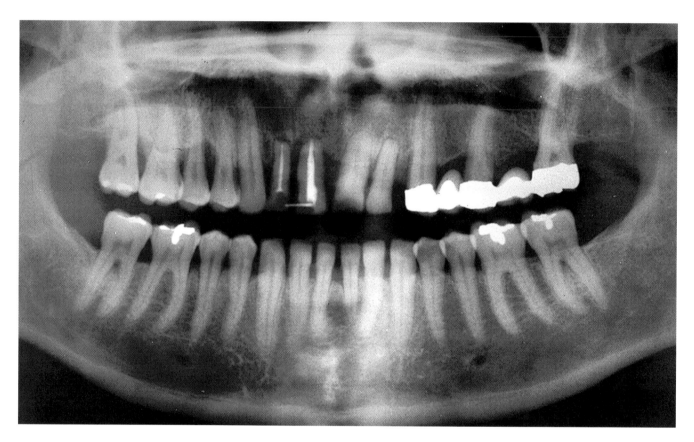

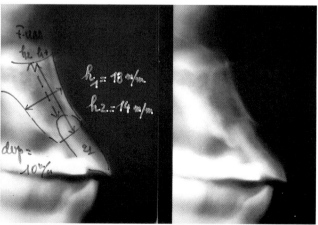

Fig 6-17 Preoperative panoramic radiograph. Implants are planned to replace the four maxillary incisors. The bone height seems sufficient. A Scanora is used to evaluate the available bone volume more precisely. The teeth, which are going to be extracted, are provisionally kept to give an indication of the ideal axis for the prosthesis. (Radiography by Dr G. Pasquet and Dr R. Cavezian.)

Fig 6-18 Same patient. Scanora view. Cross-sectional image of position 21. The bone volume is clearly visible. To the left, comments are made by the radiologist. (Radiography by Dr G. Pasquet and Dr R. Cavezian.)

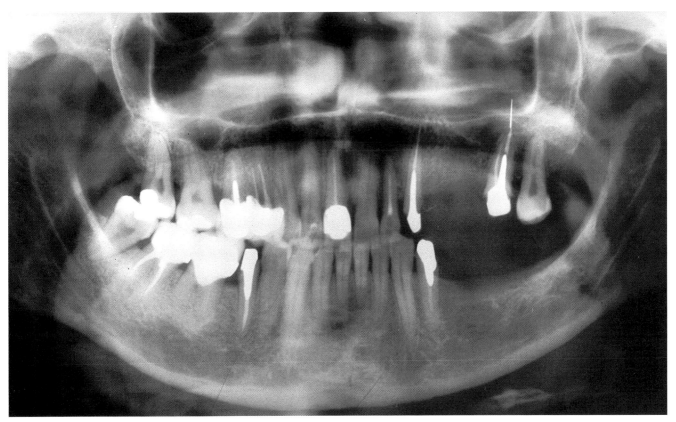

Fig 6-19 Preoperative panoramic radiograph. Implants are to be placed in the mandibular left segment. The bone height above the mandibular nerve seems satisfactory. (Radiography by Dr G. Pasquet and Dr R. Cavezian.)

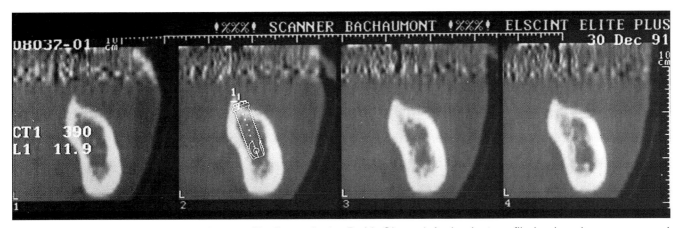

Fig 6-20 Same patient. Dentascan image. (Radiography by Dr M. Giwerc.) An implant profile is placed on a proposed implant site. Note the knife-edged ridge. A bone regeneration procedure should be considered.

Surgical Guide

The surgical guide is an indispensable tool during implant treatment. It serves as the link between the prosthetic and the surgical teams. The guide may be designed in several different manners. Two of them should be mentioned. The first is easy to fabricate but is not very precise and leaves great freedom for the surgeon. The second, on the other hand, allows previewing of any discrepancies between prosthetic and surgical demands before surgery.

Solution No. 1

Impression

Fabrication of an ideal surgical guide at the laboratory without consideration of the anatomic conditions

The surgeon judges the best surgical possibilities, as indicated by the guide

This solution is best suited for areas with large bone volume (wide crests) and for the posterior regions (Figs 6-21 to 6-26).

Figs 6-21 and 6-22 Surgical guide for placing implants in positions 44, 45, and 46. It consists of a plastic guide with ideal hole positions for the implant placement indicated.

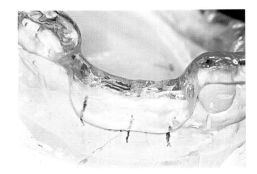
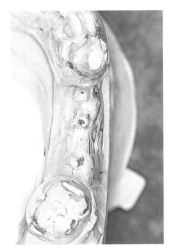

Advantages: is simple; causes little obstruction during surgery.
Disadvantages: has low precision; does not indicate the vertical orientation of the implants.

Figs 6-23 and 6-24 Surgical guide for placing implants in positions 24, 25, and 26. Only the vestibular aspects of the teeth are fabricated.

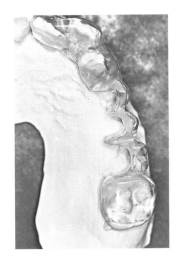
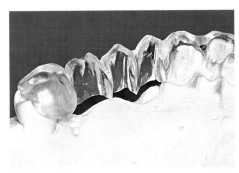

Advantages: provides good access and good visibility of the field of operation; leaves a certain freedom to the surgeon.
Disadvantage: does not provide sufficient orientation in situations where esthetics is important.

Figs 6-25 and Fig 6-26 Surgical guide for placing implants in positions 46 and 47. The teeth are completely made from a waxup. They are thereafter pierced to indicate the ideal implant axis and position.

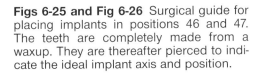
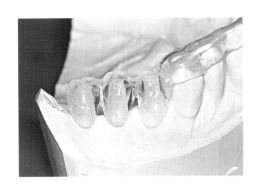

Advantages: is very direct; suits all indications when it comes to ideal placement.
Disadvantage: is sometimes bulky; leaves little visibility for the surgeon during drilling.

Solution No. 2

Impression

Fabrication of a radiographic guide at the laboratory with positioning of radiographic markers for an objective judgment of the prosthetic limitations

Scanner procedure (evaluation of the useful bone volume)

Modification of the radiographic guide into a precise surgical guide

The surgeon follows the exact indications of the guide

This protocol is preferable for solutions with high esthetic demands (Figs 6-27 to 6-31).

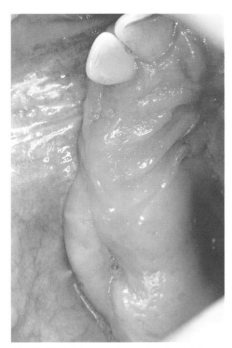

Fig 6-27 Initial clinical situation. Three or four implants are planned for the maxillary right segment.

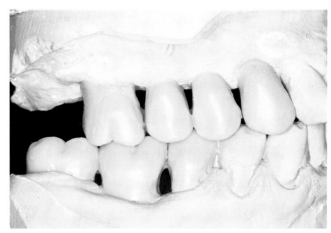

Fig 6-28 Same patient. Presurgical waxup.

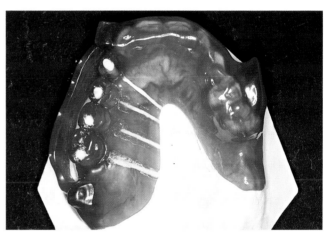

Fig 6-29 Same patient. From the waxup, a radiographic guide is made at the laboratory. The ideal orientations of the implants are indicated through the guide. A radiopaque material (gutta-percha, zinc phosphate cement, etc) is placed in the holes. The patient wears this guide during the scanning.

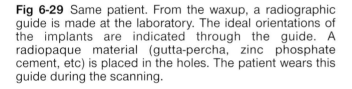

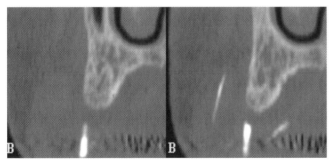

Fig 6-30 Same patient. Dentascan image. Note the visualization of the ideal prosthetic axis. Depending on available bone volume, the orientation can be modified. In the case presented, the drilling should be done somewhat more palatally.

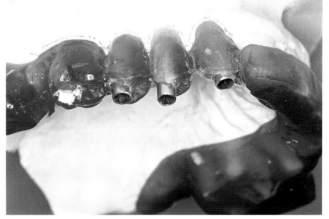

Fig 6-31 Same patient. Final surgical guide. Depending on the information obtained from the scanning, the orientation of the markers is modified. The guide is then sterilized and delivered to the surgeon. (Prostheses by Dr J.-M. Gonzalez, Dr P. Rajzbaum, X. Daniel, and P. Poussin.) (Radiography by Dr N. Bellaïche.)

Treatment Sequence

It is possible to adapt the treatment sequence to fit the clinical situation. The different alternatives are selected based on the following parameters:

- Patient's health condition
- Presence or absence of keratinized mucosa
- Bone density
- Number and relative position of implants
- Plaque control conditions
- Stability of the transitional prosthesis

Option 1 (standard protocol)
1. Stage 1 surgery (implant insertion)
2. Healing phase (3 to 6 months) + provisionalization
3. Stage 2 surgery (placement of healing abutment)
4. Final abutment placement
5. Impression for the final prosthesis

Option 2 (one-stage surgery)
1. Stage 1 surgery (implant insertion) + placement of healing abutment
2. Healing phase (3 to 6 months) + provisionalization
3. Final abutment placement
4. Impression for the final prosthesis

Option 3 (standard protocol with impression at stage 1 surgery)
1. Stage 1 surgery + impression
2. Healing phase (3 to 6 months) + provisionalization
3. Stage 2 surgery + placement of final abutments (TiAdapt) + provisional acrylic resin prosthesis
4. Impression for the final prosthesis

Option 4 (one-stage surgery with impression at stage 1 surgery)
1. Stage 1 surgery + impression + placement of healing abutments
2. Healing phase (3 to 6 months) + provisionalization
3. Placement of final abutments (TiAdapt) + provisional acrylic resin prosthesis
4. Impression for the final prosthesis

Option 5 (immediate loading)
1. Stage 1 surgery + placement of final abutments
2. Gingival healing (10 days)
3. Impression for the final prosthesis

Note

There is not enough clinical data to allow sufficient evaluation and selection of option No. 5 in routine practice. Today, this indication is reserved for the anterior segment of the mandible in patients without parafunctional habits or signs of bruxism.

	Option 1 Standard protocol	Option 2 One-stage protocol	Option 3 Standard protocol + impression at stage 1	Option 4 One-stage protocol + impression at stage 1	Option 5 Immediate-loading protocol
Advantage	Well known and predictable protocol. Few problems with provisionalization.	Cost reduction and simplification of treatment. One less surgical intervention.	Simplification of treatment. Few problems with provisionalization. Placement of provisional prosthesis at stage 2 surgery.	Cost reduction and simplification of treatment. Reduction of treatment time. One less surgical intervention.	Cost reduction and simplification of treatment. Reduction of treatment time.
Disadvantage	Two surgical interventions. Risk for cover screw exposure in thin gingiva.	Need for excellent primary implant stability.	Prolonged surgical duration. Two surgical interventions. Risk for cover screw exposure in thin gingiva.	Need for excellent primary implant stability. Prolonged surgical duration.	Lack of clinical data.
Indications	All.	Posterior segments.	Esthetic segments.	Posterior segments.	Mandibular symphysis.
General contraindication	Patients with general pathoses and relative contraindications to local anesthesia. Hyperanxious patients.	Patients with poor plaque control. Patients with risk for local infections. Need for bone regeneration procedures.	Patients with general pathoses and relative contraindications to local anesthesia. Hyperanxious patients.	Patients with poor plaque control. Patients with risk for local infections. Need for bone regeneration procedures.	Patients with poor plaque control. Patients with risk for local infections.
Local contraindication	None.	Sharp bone crest. Little or no kera-tinized gingiva. Poor primary implant stability. Unstable provisional prosthesis.	None.	Sharp bone crest. Little or no kera-tinized gingiva. Poor primary implant stability. Unstable provisional prosthesis.	Implants shorter than 13 mm. Fewer than six fixtures. Type III and IV bone.

Summary: Indications for one-stage or two-stage procedure	
Two-stage procedure	**One-stage procedure**
Systemic disease	Wide crest
Smoking	Large area of keratinized gingiva
Low bone density (Type III-IV) Low bone-healing potential (BHP 2-3)	Dense bone with thick cortical layers
Need for bone crest augmentation	Good plaque control
Periodontal risk factors	Stable transitional prosthesis

Surgical Technique

In the posterior regions, the surgeon has to place implants in bone with very diverse density. Sometimes the presence of major anatomic obstacles (eg, the inferior alveolar nerve) makes it impossible to find bicortical anchorage for obtaining good primary implant stability.

Also, certain implant indications cannot be pursued because of the risk of placing the implants in too limited space. This is particularly true for the replacement of the maxillary lateral incisors or the mandibular central incisors.

This is the reason for the development of implants with larger and smaller diameters. However, the increased number of different implants results in more operative decisions. The surgeon has to adapt the drilling sequence, not only to each implant diameter but also to each type of bone density (Figs 6-32 and 6-33).

For each patient, there is an appropriate sequence of drilling. However, there are no absolute rules. For example, drills with larger diameters are not always used throughout the complete depth of the site. Likewise, the drilling depth of the countersink should be adapted to each clinical situation.

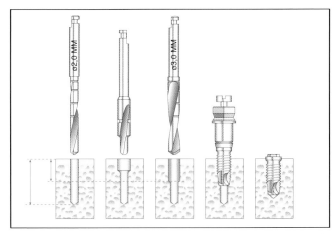

Fig 6-32 Drilling sequence in low-density bone (Type IV). The sites are not enlarged to their full depth with the last drill. This makes it possible to increase the initial stability of the implant.

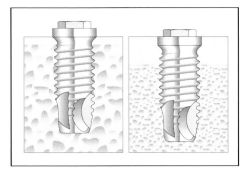

Fig 6-33 An ideal countersinking of the implant related to bone density. In soft Type IV bone (left), it is preferable not to widen the site too much to allow a firm seating in the cortical bone.

Note
Self-tapping implants are recommended in high-density bone. For soft bone, it is preferable to use implants with less tapping performance.

Note
When the bone in the posterior mandible is very dense, the use of a wide implant may lead to marginal bone resorption during the healing period. It seems preferable to avoid the use of Wide Platform implants in Type I bone.

Note
The denser the bone, the greater the risk of overheating, and the drilling should be carefully handled under ample irrigation.

Proposal for drilling sequences as a function of implant diameter and bone density

Bone Density	Round bur	Twist drill (2-mm)	Pilot drill (2 to 3-mm)	Twist drill (2.4-mm)	Twist drill (2.8-mm)	Counter-sink NP	Screw tap NP	Twist drill (3-mm)	Counter-sink RP	Twist drill (3.35-mm)	Twist drill (3.7-mm)	Screw tap RP	Twist drill (3.85-mm)	Screw tap WP	Manual wrench
Narrow platform (3.3-mm)															
Low	+	+		+		+									
Medium	+	+			+	+									
High	+	+			+	+	+								
Regular platform (3.75-mm)															
Low	+	+	+		+				+						
Medium	+	+	+					+	+						
High	+	+	+					+	+	+/−		+			
Regular platform (4-mm)															
Low	+	+	+					+	+						
Medium	+	+	+					+	+	+		+/−			
High	+	+	+					+	+		+	+	+/−		+/−
Wide platform (5-mm)															
Low	+	+	+					+	+		+/−				
Medium	+	+	+					+	+				+		+
High	+	+	+					+	+				+	+	+
Wide platform (5.5-mm)															
Low	+	+	+					+	+		+/−				
Medium	+	+	+					+	+				+	+/−	+
High	+	+	+					+	+				+	+	+

Advanced Surgical Techniques

Inadequate useful bone volume often represents a relative or absolute contraindication to implant placement. There are, however, many protocols available for bone augmentation, such as guided tissue regeneration and bone grafting.

Guided Tissue Regeneration

Guided tissue regeneration is used to increase the width of the bone crest and sometimes to increase the vertical dimensions. The principle is based on the creation of an artificial space between a barrier membrane and the bone. The blood clot will then only be in contact with osteogenic cells, which will regenerate new bone in the protected area. In original protocol, the membranes were used without any space filler, and the shape of the void between bone and membrane was maintained via mechanical reinforcements to the membrane (titanium frames, space screws, etc). However, it has been demonstrated that it is preferable that bone be placed under the membrane for scaffolding. Bone chips gathered during drilling or fragments of bone harvested from other areas in the mouth are useful.

> **Note**
> No provisional prosthesis should be placed in contact with the operated area for a minimum of 3 weeks.

The guided tissue regeneration procedure may be performed according to different protocols:
- One-stage: Bone regeneration starts at the time of implant placement.
- Two-stage: Bone regeneration surgery is followed by 8 months' healing before implant surgery.

One-stage protocol (Figs 6-34 to 6-36)

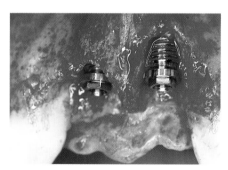 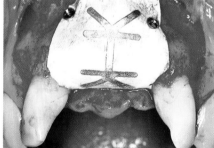 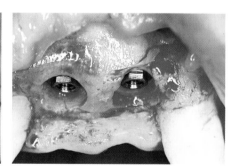

Fig 6-34 The patient has lost teeth 11 and 21 to trauma. Note the loss of the labial bone plates. Note the exposure of part of the implants.

Fig 6-35 Same patient. A nonresorbable membrane (Gore-Tex with titanium reinforcement) is placed above the bone defect. The membrane is stabilized with the aid of microscrews (Nolwenn System).

Fig 6-36 Same patient. After 8 months of healing, the membrane is removed. Note the complete coverage of the implant threads. (The final clinical situation is presented in chapter 4, Figs 4-39 to 4-44.)

Two-stage protocol (Figs 6-37 to 6-41)

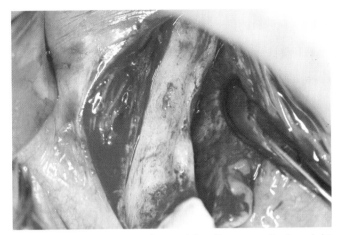

Fig 6-37 Implants are planned for the mandibular right segment. The crest is too knife-edged sharp for implant placement under favorable conditions.

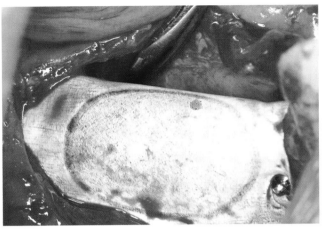

Fig 6-38 Same patient. A nonresorbable membrane (Gore-Tex) covers the crest. It is kept apart from the bone with spacer screws. No material is placed between the bone and the membrane.

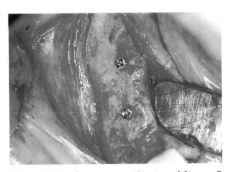

Fig 6-39 Same patient. After 8 months, an enlargement of the crest of about 5 mm has been obtained.

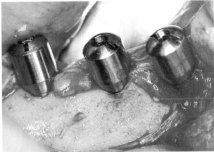

Fig 6-40 Same patient at second-stage surgery after 4 months healing. Note the corticalization of the bone.

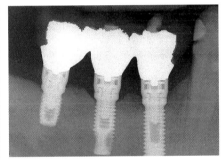

Fig 6-41 Same patient at follow-up 3 years after loading. (Prostheses by Dr J.-M. Gonzalez, Dr P. Rajzbaum, and C. Laval.)

Technical note

If only a few threads of the implant are exposed, it is possible to cover the dehiscence without membrane.

Autogenous bone grafting

The grafting techniques applied to implant treatment have been borrowed from maxillofacial reconstruction procedures. The corresponding protocols are well defined and the results are predictable.

The grafts may be taken from the chin, the hip, or the skull (Fig 6-42). Autogenous sinus grafts have a sufficiently high success rate to be considered as a routine procedure.

Most grafting protocols prescribe 6 months of healing before implant placement (Figs 6-43 to 6-47). There are some indications for a simultaneous grafting and implant procedure, but the predictability remains with the two-stage technique.

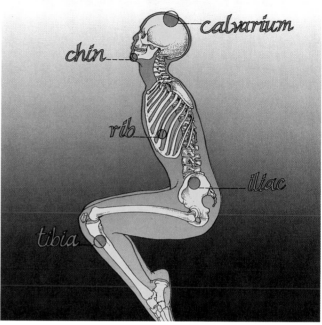

Fig 6-42 Different donor sites for bone surgery. Only the cranial plates, the chin, and the iliac crest can be used by the maxillofacial surgeon. (Drawing by Merry Scheitlin.)

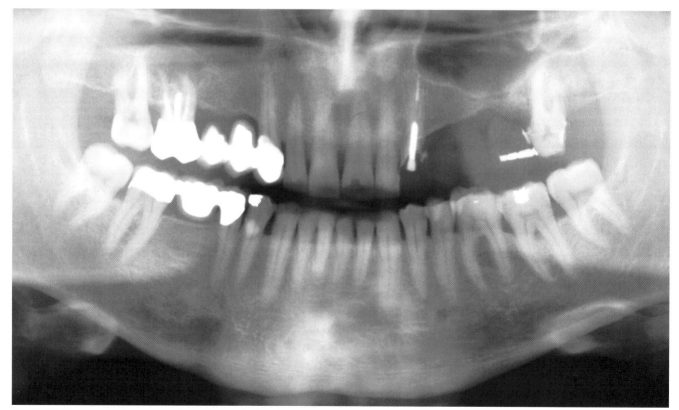

Fig 6-43 Presurgical panoramic radiograph. Implants are to be placed in the maxillary left segment. Note the low height of the bone crest. (Radiography by Dr G. Pasquet and Dr R. Cavezian.)

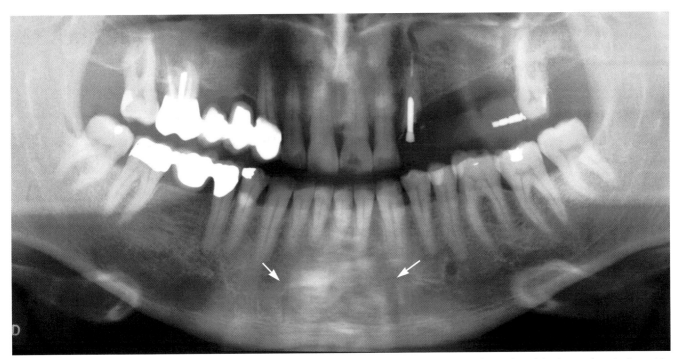

Fig 6-44 Same patient. A bone graft with both cortical and cancellous bone is taken from the chin *(arrow)* and placed in the sinus cavity. Six months of healing is recommended before the implants are placed. (Radiography by Dr G. Pasquet and Dr R. Cavezian.)

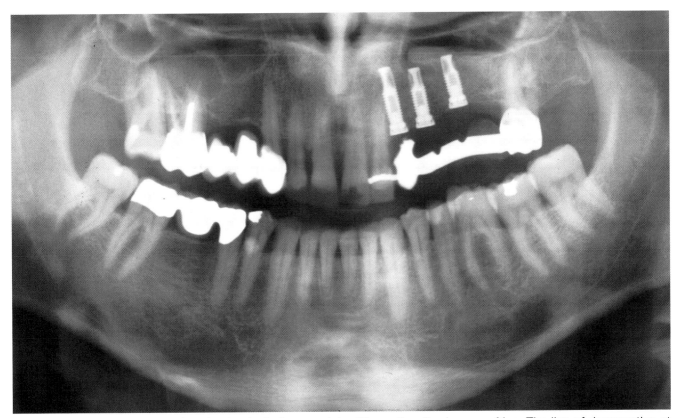

Fig 6-45 Same patient 6 months after implant placement, ie, 12 months after bone grafting. The line of demarcation at the donor site in the chin has disappeared. (Radiography by Dr G. Pasquet and Dr R. Cavezian.)

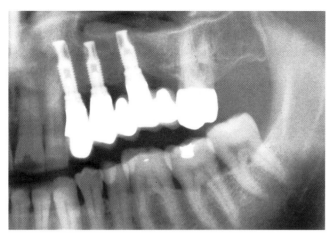

Fig 6-46 Same patient 2 years after loading of the prosthesis. Note the stability of the bone level around the implants. (Radiography by Dr G. Pasquet and Dr R. Cavezian.)

Note
No provisional prosthesis should be placed in contact with the operated area for a minimum of 3 weeks.

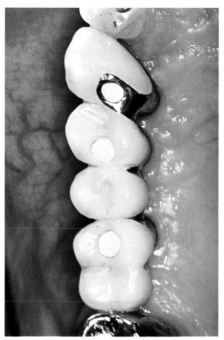

Fig 6-47 Same patient. Occlusal view. (Prosthesis by Dr D. Lebreton and S. Tissier.)

Postoperative Follow-up and Maintenance

Follow-up of the patient after the therapeutic phase is part of successful treatment. When the surgeon and prosthodontist are different persons, it is important to define who is responsible for the patient's follow-up after the prosthetic procedures are finalized.

The patient is seen at 8 to 10 days after implant placement for removal of the sutures. If the healing is satisfactory, the prosthesis may then be rebased. (If grafting or bone regeneration procedures have been implemented, it is necessary to wait a minimum of 6 weeks). The patient should then be examined about every 4 to 6 weeks to verify mucosal healing to detect premature exposure of the cover screws, and to rebase the prosthesis if needed.

The patient is seen 8 to 10 days after placement of the healing abutments for removal of the sutures. The final abutments are placed 4 to 6 weeks later.

Fabrication of the prosthesis may commence immediately after the placement of the final abutments. The patient is examined 15 days after the prosthesis is delivered.

Screw-retained prostheses

Note
The repeated loosening of a gold screw represents an alarm signal (see chapter 3, page 53). It should not be retightened until the cause of the problem has been identified.

Cemented prostheses

The prosthesis stability is checked. Peri-implant tissue health is carefully evaluated, because cement could remain under the mucosa and lead to inflammation. In the absence of signs of inflammation, the patient is recalled at 3 months, 6 months, and then one or two times per year.

Note

This technique refers to CeraOne, CerAdapt, and TiAdapt abutments. The procedure starts with the tightening of the abutment gold alloy screws. The tightening should be performed with the electric control instrument and countertorque (different torque values for different platforms; see table on page 55). It is imperative that proper components are used and that the tightening procedure be performed correctly, to ensure the full tension of the screws. This is the final tightening of the screws; loosening cannot be checked after cementation, and alarm signals, such as screw loosening, are difficult to identify. Temporary cementation is not a solution for retrievability, because the long-term stability of the cement junction is not predictable.

Due to these limitations, this option is only recommended for situations where the biomechanical risk factors are low (see chapter 3). It is also important to ensure a firm cement bond, because if it dissolves or breaks for one abutment it might not be detected but will lead to an unfavorable distribution of force.

At the periodic follow-up visits, the practitioner should do the following:

- Take a radiograph with an orthogonal view to check for possible bone resorption.
- Evaluate the health condition of the peri-implant mucosa by checking:
  - Sulcular bleeding (Note: The probing force should not be too strong, because the soft tissue junction to the implant is weaker than the periodontal attachment).
  - Peri-implant mucosal inflammation (mucositis).
- Test the prosthesis stability. If the prosthesis is perceived to be stable, the screw tightening should not be checked unnecessarily.
- Verify the occlusion.

If peri-implant mucosal inflammation is found, the following is suggested:

- Ensure that the prosthesis allows good oral hygiene.
- Check the patient's plaque control capacity.
- Look for possible sites of periodontal inflammation that might be the origin of the problem.

After the probable etiology of the inflammation is eliminated, the patient should be examined at 3 months. If the symptoms persist, a more advanced periodontal and peri-implant examination should be performed.

Suggested readings

Surgical guide

Assemat-Tessandier X, Sansemat JJ. Proposition de guide chirurgical dans la technique des prothèses sur implants ostéo-intégrés de Brånemark. Cah Proth 1990;6:77-87.

Gonzalez JM, Giraud L. L'évaluation préchirurgicale en implantologie. Réalités Clin 1992;3:283-291.

Bone density

Lekholm U, Zarb GA. Patient selection and preparation. In: Brånemark P-I, Zarb GA, Albrektsson T (eds). Tissue-Integrated Prostheses: Osseointegration in Clinical Dentistry. Chicago: Quintessence, 1985.

Jaffin R, Berman C. The excessive loss of Brånemark fixtures in type IV bone: A 5-year analysis. J Periodontol 1991;62:2-4.

Rothman SLG. Dental Applications of Computerized Tomography: Surgical Planning for Implant Placement. Chicago: Quintessence, 1998.

One-stage surgery

Bernard JP, Belser UC, Martinet JP, Borgis SA. Osseointegration of Brånemark fixtures using a single-step operating technique. A preliminary prospective one-year study in the edentulous mandible. Clin Oral Implants Res 1995;6:122-129.

Collaert B, De Bruyn H. Comparison of Brånemark fixture integration and short-term survival using one-stage or two-stage surgery in completely and partially edentulous mandibles. Clin Oral Implants Res 1998;9:131-135.

Ericsson I, Randow K, Glantz PO, Lindhe J, Nilner K. Clinical and radiographical features of submerged and non-submerged titanium implants. Clin Oral Implants Res 1994;5:185-189.

Self-tapping implants

Friberg B, Nilson H, Olsson M, Palmquist C. MKII. The self-tapping Brånemark implant: The 5-year results of a prospective 3-center study. Clin Oral Implants Res 1997;8:279-285.

Bone density evaluation during implant placement

Friberg B, Sennerby L, Roos J, Lekholm U. Identification of bone quality in conjunction with insertion of titanium implants. A pilot study in jaw autopsy specimens. Clin Oral Implants Res 1995;6:213-219.

Wide diameter implants

Langer B, Langer L, Herrmann I, Jörnéus L. The wide fixture: A solution for special bone situations and a rescue for a compromised implant. Part 1. Int J Oral Maxillofac Implants 1993;8:400-408.

Renouard F, Robert P, Godard L, Fievet C. Risk factors in implant surgical procedures: Wide diameter implants, bone regeneration and tobacco use. J Parodontol Implant Orale. 1998;17:299-314.

Implant placement protocol

Slaughter T, Babbush C, Langer B, Buser D, Holmes R. Solutions for specific bone situations: Should we use different implant designs for different bone? Should we use different surgical approaches for different bone using the same implant? Int J Oral Maxillofac Implants 1994;9:19-29.

Impression at implant level

Kupeyan HK, Brien RL. The role of the implant impression in abutment selection: A technical note. Int J Oral Maxillofac Implants 1995;10:429-433.

Prestipino V, Ingber A. Implant fixture position registration at the time of fixture placement surgery. Pract Periodont Aesthet Dent 1992;5:1-7.

Guided Bone Regeneration

Buser D, Dahlin C, Schenk RK. Guided Bone Regeneration in Implant Dentistry. Chicago: Quintessence, 1994.

Simion M, Jovanovic SA, Trisi P, Scarano A, Piattelli A. Vertical ridge augmentation around dental implants using a membrane technique and autogenous bone or allografts in humans. Int J Periodont Rest Dent 1998;18:9-23.

Additional readings

Beumer J, Lewis SG. The Brånemark Implant System: Clinical and Laboratory Procedures. St Louis: Ishiyaku EuroAmerica, 1989.

Cavezian R, Pasquet G. Imagerie et diagnostic en odonto-stomatologie. Paris: Masson, 1988.

Gröndahl K, Ekestubbe A, Gröndahl HG. Radiography in Oral Endosseous Prosthetics. Göteborg: Nobel Biocare, 1996.

Jensen O. The Sinus Bone Graft. Chicago: Quintessence, 1998.

Lacan A, Michelin J, Dana A, Levy L, Meyer D. Nouvelle Imagerie Dentaire. Paris: CDP, 1993.

Patient Relations

A meeting of about 20 dentists was organized to discuss the theme of communication. During the meeting, the following question was put forward: "How can one give confidence to a patient who is afraid of experiencing pain during or after implant surgery? Can one convince the patient that placement of implants is not painful?"

After some pondering, participants gave several answers:

- The patient will be fine, because he or she will receive medication to prevent the pain.
- This surgery is less painful than wisdom tooth extraction.
- Before placement of the implants, a computerized tomographic scan is made to confirm the indication.
- This problem should be discussed with the surgeon

The practitioners present at this meeting had already treated one to five patients with implant-supported prostheses. They were then asked if, according to their experience, any of the patients had complained about pain during or after the treatment. After a while, the practitioners admitted that all patients had been pleasantly surprised about how little pain and how few postoperative problems they had experienced.

This discussion revealed that the problem of communication with the patient is not the lack of information or knowledge, but rather the practitioner's inability to analyze and use this understanding in an effective way. Although they had treated implant patients, they had not reflected on or prepared for an answer to this important question: "Does implant surgery hurt?"

Good communication is indispensable in the practitioner's relationship with the patient—not to have the ability to convince at any price and make sure that the patient chooses to receive implants, but to better understand the patient's demands and respond to his or her uncertainties.

Proposal 1: Communicate = Listen

To acquire the ability to motivate a patient for a treatment that is perceived, first and foremost, as painful, expensive, and difficult, the clinician must have thoroughly considered the problem and have formulated an appropriate response to the patient's concerns.

The practitioner should not impose a treatment; he or she should justify it. Therefore, the practitioner must take time to get to know the patient and understand his or her motivation. To establish a good relationship with the patient, the clinician must first define the pertinent areas of concern and thereafter the technicalities. Discussing these matters around a desk is a better means of building confidence and creating a good relationship between patient and practitioner.

Note: It is important to reserve time outside the technical environment to allow for the patient to build confidence.

Proposal 2: Communicate = Prepare

During the consultation before implant treatment, the patients almost always ask the same questions. It is important to have reflected on these questions and have prepared answers to be able to give a truthful and encouraging response.

The concerns of patients can generally be condensed into six inquiries:

- Does it hurt?
- How long will the implants last?
- I have a friend who received six and has already lost five.
- Does it really work with synthetic materials?
- How much does it cost? It appears to be very expensive.
- Aren't they rejected sometimes?

Does it hurt?

The implants are placed in an atraumatic manner and the bone is handled gently to reduce the risk of failure. All sequences of the operation are performed very smoothly, somewhat like microsurgery. The intervention is much less traumatic then the extraction of a wisdom tooth. The only aftereffect is associated with the loosened gingiva and swelling should be expected, in an intensity that varies with the patient. Pain relief medication is generally not needed for more than 1 day.

How long will the implants last?

Statistically, the implants could be retained for the rest of the recipient's life. The success rate is between 90% and 99% depending on the clinical situation. The implant-supported prosthesis can be considered as natural teeth and will react in a similar manner. Occlusal overload may lead to material fracture, and poor oral hygiene entails an increased risk of tissue inflammation around the implants. Regular dental examinations are mandatory.

I have a friend who received six and has already lost five.

There are a number of implant types, the vast majority of which have not been subjected to any clinical study. Selection of a reliable system is crucial.

However, before implant treatment is planned, a number of different clinical parameters must be evaluated, especially the condition of the bone. It is not until all these factors are considered that it can be determined whether implant treatment is an option.

Does it really work with synthetic materials?

The only studies that have been satisfactorily performed to affirm long-term reliability of a synthetic material for integration with bone have been conducted on commercially pure titanium. Other materials should be considered experimental.

How much does it cost?

The cost of this treatment is generally still on a high level. Yet, most often, it is at the same level as are conventional fixed restorations but with proven, high, long-term reliability. A serious financial evaluation should be performed before treatment commences. However, sometimes it is necessary to wait for the preimplant examination (computerized tomographic scan, dental cast, etc) to be able to make the final cost evaluation.

Aren't they rejected sometimes?

There is no immunologic rejection of titanium implants. Commercially pure titanium is perfectly biocompatible and is accepted by the organism. This does not mean that it has a 100% success rate, but a failure is manifested as light mobility and a sensitivity around the implant. The implant is removed in such situations and may be replaced with another implant of the same size after healing.

Inflammatory reactions (osteitis) leading to substantial pain are extremely rare.

Proposal 3: Communicate = Adapt

Words and phrases do not have the same meaning to all people. Thus, the word *car* could mean, for different people:

- Utility car
- Sports car
- Antique (classic) car

A great number of parameters influence the comprehension of the verbal input for even such simple and apparently objective a word as car. Experience, financial means, the need for affirmation, or on the contrary, isolation, and a number of other factors makes the spontaneous and unconscious interpretation of a word vary from one individual to another.

If the word *car* may allow such different perceptions, then think about the words *implant*, *surgery*, *osseointegration*, *periodontal disease*, and so on. When a practitioner talks for the first time to a patient about the possibility of using implants, the patient will unconsciously translate *implant* into one of the following words:

- *Money*
- *Surgery*
- *Operating room*
- *Pain*
- *Comfort*
- *Rejection*
- *Failure*
- *Hopeless prosthesis*

The patient certainly will not think: "a titanium screw, 3.75 mm in diameter and 10 mm in length, that may host 7 different types of abutment, especially the well-known CerAdapt, which would be so well indicated in my particular situation."

In spite of the limited time available, the clinician must know the patient sufficiently to be able to use words, phrases, and expressions that will be understood. For a young patient (35 years) who works in the stock market, is living in the present, and is motivated by success and profits, it is not worthwhile to explain that the implants have been developed over the last 50 years in Göteborg, Sweden, starting at a small laboratory. On the other hand, this explanation might reassure a considerably older, insecure patient, who is worrying about the future, turning to the past, and more conservative.

This appreciation of the different personalities of patients is difficult to gain rapidly, but it is necessary for the practitioner who wishes to communicate and not only listen but also understand.

Suggested readings

De Bruyn H, Collaert B, Linden U, Björn AL. Patient's opinion and treatment outcome of fixed rehabilitation on Brånemark implants: A 3-year follow-up study in private dental practices. Clin Oral Implants Res 1997;8:265-271.

Rozencweig D. Des clés pour réussir au cabinet dentaire. Paris: Quintessence International, 1998.

Chapter 8

Complications

First-Stage Surgery

Problem	Possible Causes	Solutions
Hemorrhage during drilling	Lesion or injury of an artery	The implant placement will stop the bleeding.
Implant mobility after placement	Soft bone Imprecise preparation	Remove the implant and replace with one of larger diameter. If the mobility is small, prolong the healing time.
Exposed implant threads	Too-narrow crest	Cover the threads with coagulum or place a membrane.
Swelling lingually directly after implant placement at the mandibular symphysis	Incision of an artery branch sublingually	Emergency: Send the patient to a specialist center for coagulation of the artery under general anesthesia.
Substantial postoperative pain remaining after some days	Osteitis due to a too-aggressive preparation or a bacterial contamination	Remove the affected implant.
Insensitivity of the lower lip	Incision or compression of the mandibular inferior nerve	If the insensitivity persists after a week, use a CT scan to determine which implant is causing the problem and remove it.
Exposed cover screw after a few weeks	Cover screw not placed deep enough; thin mucosa	Never try to retighten the cover screw. Prescribe rigorous oral hygiene.
	Pressure on the tissue from the transitional prosthesis	Avoid the transition prosthesis.
Abscess around a cover screw after a few weeks	Implant is not integrating (low probability)	Remove the implant.
	Infection around the cover screw (which often is a little loose)	Make a flap, remove the granulation tissue, disinfect with chlorhexidine, change the cover screw, and resuture.

173

Second-Stage Surgery + Abutment Connection

Problem	Possible Causes	Solutions
Slightly sensitive but perfectly immobile implant	Imperfect osseointegration	Cover the implant for 2 to 3 months and test again.
Slightly painful and mobile implant	Lack of integration	Remove the implant.
Difficulty inserting a transfer screw, gold screw, or healing cap	Damaged inner thread of abutment screw	Change the abutment screw.
Inability to perfectly connect the abutment to the implant	Insufficient bone milling	Place a local anesthesia, use a bone mill with guide, remove the bone, clean with saline solution, and replace the abutment.
Granulation tissue around the implant head	Traumatic placement of the implant; compression from the transition prosthesis; a lid above the cover screw	Open the area and disinfect with chlorhexidine. If the lesion is too large, consider a bone regeneration or grafting technique.

Prosthetic Procedure; Control After Prosthesis Placement

Problem	Possible Causes	Solutions
Pain or sensation when tightening gold screws (during try-in of prosthesis)	Misfit between prosthesis and abutments	Cut the prosthesis, interlock the pieces, and solder the prosthesis at the laboratory. Retry the prosthesis.
Loosening of one or more prosthetic screws at the first inspection after 2 week	Occlusal problem	Retighten, verify the occlusion, and recheck after 2 weeks.
Loosening of prosthetic screws at the second check or later	Occlusal problem or misfit between prosthesis and abutments	Verify the occlusion and/or the prosthetic fit.
	Too-large extension	Reduce the extension.
	Unfavorable prosthetic concept	Change the prosthetic design (add an implant, etc). In all cases, change the prosthetic screws.
Abscess close to an implant	Poor fit of the abutment to the implant	Verify the abutment fit with a radiograph. Remove the abutment, sterilize it, remove the granulation tissue, disinfect with chlorhexidine, and replace the abutment.
Development of pain after placement of the prosthesis	Disintegration of an implant	Remove the implant.
	Peri-implant infection	See below
Fracture of a prosthetic screw or an abutment screw	Occlusal problem, lack of fit between prosthesis and abutment or unfavorable prosthetic design	If the occlusion or the adaptation of the prosthesis seems right, modify the prosthetic design (reduce or eliminate extensions, reduce the width of occlusal surfaces, reduce cuspal inclination, add implants, etc).

Fracture of veneering material	Occlusal problem	Verify the occlusion.
	Bruxism or parafunction	Make a nightguard.
Fracture of the framework	Weak metal frame end or too-large extension	Remake the prosthesis; modify the prosthetic design (reduce or eliminate extensions, reduce width and height of occlusal surfaces, reduce cusp inclination, add implants, etc).
	Bruxism or parafunction	Make a nightguard.
Implant fracture	Occlusal overload	Remove the implant with a special trephine drill, wait 2 to 6 months, if possible, and place a wider implant. Review the prosthetic design (place more implants, etc) and remake the prosthesis.
1. Continuing bone loss around one or more implants	Infection (peri-implantitis)	Remove the etiologic factors (poor plaque control, prosthesis geometry in relation to the mucosa, etc). Look for bacterial pockets around the natural teeth. Possibly make a bacteria test. Cut open the lesion. Adjust the peri-implant tissues (gingival graft). Consider a bone regeneration procedure.
2. Continuing bone loss around one or more implants	Occlusal overload	Modify the prosthetic design (reduce or eliminate extensions, reduce the width of occlusal surfaces, reduce cuspal inclination, add implants, etc).
Visibility of titanium abutment through the mucosa		Make a connective tissue graft under the mucosa. Change the abutment to ceramic material (CerAdapt).
Substantial phonetic problems that do not disappear after 2 to 3 months		Close the interimplant space (pay attention to maintenance possibilities). Make a removable gingival prosthesis. Replace the fixed prosthesis with a removable implant-supported denture.
Bleeding on probing	Mucositis or peri-implantitis	Remove etiologic factors (poor plaque control, prosthesis geometry in relation to the mucosa, etc). Look for bacterial pockets around the natural teeth. Possibly make a bacteria test. Cut open the lesion. Adjust the peri-implant tissues (gingival graft). Consider a bone regeneration procedure.

Suggested readings

Baumgarten H, Chiche G. Diagnosis and evaluation of complications and failures associated with osseointegrated implants. Compend Contin Educ Dent 1995;16:814-823.

Carlson B, Carlson GE. Prosthodontic complications in osseointegrated dental implant treatment. Int J Oral Maxillofac Implants 1994;9:90-94.

Davarpanah M, Martinez H, Kebir M, Renouard F. Complications and failures in osseointegration. J Parodontol Implant Orale 1996;15:285-314.

Friberg B, Jemt T, Lekholm U. Early failures in 4641 consecutively placed Brånemark dental implants: A study from stage 1 surgery to the connection of completed prostheses. Int J Oral Maxillofac Implants 1996;6:142-146.

Hemming KW, Schmidt A, Zarb GA. Complications and maintenance requirements for fixed prostheses and overdenture in the edentulous mandible: A 5-year report. Int J Oral Maxillofac Implants 1994;9:191-196.

Jemt T. Failures and complication in 391 consecutively inserted prostheses supported by Brånemark implants in edentulous jaws: A study of treatment from the time of prostheses placement to the first annual check-up. Int J Oral Maxillofac Implants 1991;6:270-276.

Jemt T, Lekholm U. Oral implant treatment in posterior partially edentulous jaws: A 5-year follow-up report. Int J Oral Maxillofac Implants 1993;8:635-640.

Monbelli A, van Oosten MA, Schurch E, Lang NP. The microbiata associated with successful or failing osseointegrated titanium implants. Oral Microbiol Immunol 1987;2:145-151.

Morgan MJ, James D, Robert MP. Fractures of the fixture component of an osseointegrated implant. Int J Oral Maxillofac Implants 1993;8:409-414.

Quirynen M, Naert I, van Steenberghe D, Schepers E, Calberson L, Theuniers G, et al. The cumulative failure rate of the Brånemark system in the overdenture, the fixed partial, and the fixed full prostheses design: A prospective study on 1273 fixtures. J Head Neck Pathol 1991;10:43-53.

Tolman DE, Laney WR. Tissue-integrated prosthesis complications. Int J Oral Maxillofac Implants 1991;7:477-484.